YOGA

THE ANCIENT WAY
TO HEALTH AND PEACE

Thanks to Richard Hittleman, millions of Americans practice the Eastern discipline of Yoga daily to cultivate and maintain total fitness—and to alleviate specific physical and emotional problems as well.

Don't resign yourself to the miseries of stress, obesity, poor circulation, or depression. Faithful daily application of the Yoga exercises and breathing techniques—all clearly described and illustrated with photographs in this volume—will recharge your total system and bring back the life force (prana) that's so vital to health.

Richard Hittleman's YOGA FOR TOTAL FITNESS is your path to a whole new life of joy and tranquility and maximum personal fulfillment.

RICHARD HITTLEMAN'S
YOGA FOR TOTAL FITNESS
A Bantam Book / January 1983

Photography by Thomas Burke

Models for the photographs:

Shelia Sheppard
Joseph Carter
Lisa Andante
Ruth Albee

ISBN 0-553-13812-X

Published simultaneously in the United States and Canada

Bantam Books are published by Bantam Books, Inc. Its trademark, consisting of the words "Bantam Books" and the por-
trayal of a rooster, is Registered in U.S. Patent and Trademark
Office and in other countries. Marca Registrada. Bantam
Books, Inc., 666 Fifth Avenue, New York, New York 10103.

PRINTED IN THE UNITED STATES OF AMERICA

O   0 9 8 7 6 5 4 3 2 1

RICHARD HITTLEMAN'S

YOGA
FOR TOTAL
FITNESS

Bantam Books

Toronto · New York · London · Sydney

contents

PART 2 / 137

introduction

Hatha Yoga is the most ancient and universally respected approach to holistic health. Perfected over a period of many centuries by the great spiritual teachers (**gurus**) of India, Yoga is today recognized by numerous health authorities as one of the most comprehensive systems for cultivating and maintaining a high level of physical fitness and as a series of techniques that can be effectively used in treating a variety of physical and emotional problems.

This book presents the practical applications of both these aspects of Yoga. Part 1 contains the **Fitness Programs;** Part 2 offers routines for use in special situations and to achieve specific physical objectives. During thirty years as an instructor, I have taught Yoga to several million people and have had extensive experience in the effects of the exercises (*asanas*) and breath control (*pranayama*) techniques. The programs and routines in this book are those which have consistently proven to be of great assistance in achieving the stated objectives.

Yoga proposes that cultivating genuine and lasting health of the organism requires a total approach: **all** systems of the body must receive attention. The glands, organs, ligaments, bones, joints, circulation, respiration, and so forth, are as important as the muscles that are emphasized by the majority of body-conditioning systems. In addition, a fitness program cannot be considered as complete if it neglects the health and stability of the mind and emotions. Yoga, therefore, regards body, mind, and emotions as aspects of a total entity, and its techniques are concerned with the health of each as it relates to the **whole.**

As implied above, the Yoga techniques are not to be confused with the familiar movements that comprise the various systems of calisthenics. The two are quite different. You approach the Yoga practice in a calm, serene frame of mind and perform the techniques in a series of slow, graceful, rhythmic movements that are punctuated by static **holds.** Usually, only a few repetitions are required. There is no jumping about, huffing, puffing, deliberate quickening of the heartbeat, perspiration, straining, and exhaustion. (Frequently, it is only at this point of exhaustion that the exerciser believes something has been accomplished.) People tend to confuse movement—sports, gardening, housework, and so forth—with exercise. They will say, "I get all the exercise I need with my housework and tennis." But these are the very activities that **produce** stress and tension; they cannot provide a methodical self-manipulation of the entire body, which is the Yogi's concept of total exercising. In contrast to calisthenics, **the Yoga techniques are designed to increase, not deplete, energy and life-force.**

In Yoga, we regard most conditions of ill-health and many of the symptoms of aging as unnatural. It is considered unnatural to suffer with obesity, tension, stiffness, exhaustion, nervousness, depression, respiratory conditions, congestion, deposits, poor circulation, flabbiness, headaches, and numerous other common disorders to which many people simply resign themselves. We ascribe these conditions to **improper care of the body** (through ignorance and neglect), and we offer various routines to assist in eliminating such conditions by regenerating and revitalizing the entire organism. Knowing the absolute interrelation of all parts and aspects of the organism (headaches can be caused by flat feet), we approach the resolution of all problems in a **holistic** manner. Therefore, although this book presents routines that address themselves to specific problems, we continue to emphasize that the techniques of the **Fitness Program,** as well as the Yoga nutrition principles, be given equal attention.

Because in carefully following the instructions for performing the techniques you will never experience strain, soreness or fatigue, your age and present physical condition are of minimal consequence. Indeed, the more "out of condition," stiff, weak, tense, and obese you are, the more you need the assistance that the Yoga practice offers. Such negative conditions deplete your energies, weaken the body's resistance, and pave the way for serious illnesses. You cannot experience the joy of good health nor develop your full potential when your life-force (*prana*) is continually depleted by these conditions. Hatha Yoga increases the supply of life-force and aids in maintaining it at an optimal level. This influx of additional life-force will enable you to do those things necessary for restoring the body to its proper condition.

If you are in relatively good health, your Yoga practice will not only maintain this health but will add to your strength, endurance, control, awareness, and concentration.

By faithfully practicing the **Fitness Program** (and **Special Routines**) you select, you can expect to accomplish the following:

• Strengthen and revitalize your entire body.

- Regain youthful flexibility in spine and limbs.

- Regulate and redistribute weight in accordance with your structure.

- Eliminate tension and remain alert but relaxed under pressure.

- Store life-force (*prana*) that can be released as needed.

- Acquire the ability to overcome existing negative conditions of the body, mind, and emotions.

- Increase endurance.

- Heighten resistance to many common disorders.

- Develop balance, poise, and coordination and achieve greater control of the body, mind, and emotions.

- Improve concentration and become more efficient in all of your activities.

In preparation for practice, these are the considerations:

1. Perform the techniques in a place of privacy where you will not be disturbed. A supply of fresh air is desirable.

2. You need sufficient space to stretch out on a flat surface. Cover this surface with a mat, pad, or large towel of a quiet design and color. This covering is to be used only for your practice.

3. Any clothing that is light in weight and permits complete freedom of movement is satisfactory. The less clothing, the better. Remove eyeglasses, jewelry, watch.

4. A watch or clock that allows you to read seconds should be placed in the practice area.

5. The use of a small pillow may be required for the Lotus and Head Stand.

6. At least 90 minutes must elapse after eating before you begin practice.

Patience, control, poise, rhythm, and concentration are maintained at all times during the practice session. Regard yourself as a dancer, performing a series of beautiful ballet movements in slow motion. As you continue to envision yourself in these terms, the body will be accordingly transformed.

Your initial proficiency in performing the techniques is unimportant. No two body structures are identical, so there are no standards for achievement and nothing that is competitive in Yoga. You progress entirely at your own pace and, according to your structure and physical condition, you will benefit in an immediate and direct way from whatever you are able to do. A stretch, bend, or lift of only a few inches will be of significant value. Most beginners are surprised at how quickly their bodies adjust to the positions and at the rapidity of their advancement. Patience and regular practice are the major requirements.

Always remain aware of the **progressive** nature of the practice. You will be making major changes in your body. On certain days you will experience excellent progress; on others there may be a temporary setback until your body adjusts to the new patterns. For various reasons, some areas will respond more slowly and this may make you believe that you are not progressing, or that you are even sliding backward. But a backward step is actually an element of the progressive sequence and is experienced universally among students. If, on those days when you feel such a setback occurring, you do not become discouraged but continue to practice easily and patiently (straining will only prolong the setback), within a day or two you will once again be moving ahead. Understand that a setback will probably periodically occur; it is part of the pattern.

If you are under professional care, or are uncertain of the type of movements in which you should engage, consult your physician before beginning the practice. An ever-increasing number of physicians and those in the field of health care are recommending Yoga to their patients. All of the techniques described in this book are suited for both male and female.

Yoga is a mental as well as a physical practice. The effectiveness of the techniques is increased if your mind remains fully focused on the movements, and you attempt to become acutely aware of how each is affecting the body. Gradually, you will perceive that it is not "you" performing a routine of movements, but that the movements are flowing through "you." This is a point at which the ego is transcended, and Yoga is no longer physical or mental but rather a spiritual practice.

By judicious use of the techniques in this book, you will soon come to recognize the extraordinary value of Yoga, and you will understand why it has endured these many centuries. History seems to indicate that long after the currently popular physical health fads and spiritual "awareness" systems have faded and

11

new ones have come and gone (as they do more and more frequently), Yoga will prevail. It is a total wholistic system addressing all aspects of the individual's development, and to those who devote themselves seriously, it offers the greatest of all riches: health and peace.

Richard Hittleman

part 1

the basic techniques

These are the seventeen basic *asanas* in the **Fitness Programs** and together with additional techniques, they are applied in special situations and to physical problems. Although, depending upon your time and certain other considerations, you may not be using all of these *asanas,* it is recommended that you become familiar with each of them before selecting a **Fitness Program** or undertaking the application of the **Special Routines.** Having a comprehensive, working knowledge of the different movements and **holds,** and the effect that these produce, will enable you to make an effective decision as to how the Yoga practice can be of the greatest personal service.

You can gain this recommended, working knowledge by spending your first one to two weeks of practice sessions performing the exercises in consecutive order. Each day, do as many as your time permits; at the next practice session, begin where you previously left off. In this way, you should be able to go through the cycle of the seventeen *asanas* at least seven times. Once this has been accomplished, you will be in a good position to determine which **Fitness Program** and which of the special application routines can be advantageously incorporated into your daily life.

The techniques are presented in standing, seated, and lying sequence. The instructions and photographs should be very carefully studied, since it is essential that you correctly learn and practice each movement. You should feel that you are performing an *asana* to the best of your ability before proceeding to the next. The *Notes* present important additional information about the *asanas* and the *Do not* photographs are composites of the most common mistakes made by beginning students. During the learning period, you should continue to glance at these photographs to be certain that you are not committing any of the depicted errors.

The *asanas* will become lifelong friends. If you make it a point to remain sensitive to what occurs during your Yoga practice, you will discover that each time the *asanas* are performed there is something new experienced. Your constant objective should be

15

precision: focus your total attention on what you are doing and strive to be precise, both in the execution of the movements and in counting the seconds that are indicated for the **holds.** Nothing in the instructions is arbitrary; each direction has been carefully formulated to enable you to derive the maximum benefit.

(1) complete breath

(A) standing

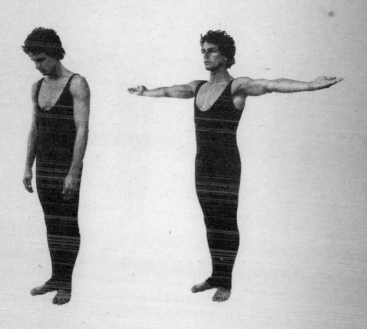

1 Stand with feet together and arms at sides. Relax. Exhale slowly and completely through nose.

  Contract abdomen to assist in complete exhalation.

2 Begin a slow inhalation through nose. Simultaneously, begin to raise arms with palms facing up.

  Push abdomen out (distend) to assist in filling lower lungs.

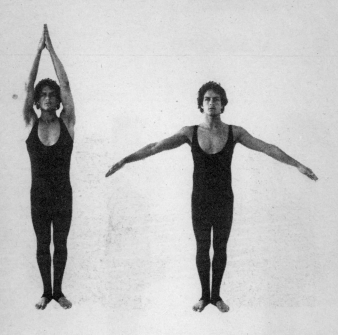

3 Continue the slow inhalation and the simultaneous raising of arms. Contract abdomen slightly and expand chest fully to assist in filling the upper part of lungs.

Palms touch overhead. Lungs should be filled at this point.

Hold position and retain air for a count of 5 (approximate seconds).

4 Execute a slow, controlled exhalation during which you slowly return arms to sides (palms down).

Relax chest during first half of exhalation; contract abdomen during second half to assist in complete emptying of lungs.

Without pause, repeat.

Perform 5 times during learning period.

(B) seated

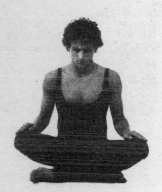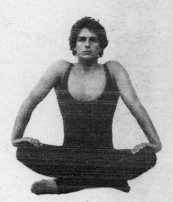

5 Sit on your mat in a simple cross legged position. Draw legs in as far as possible. Palms rest on thighs. Spine must be held straight.

Exhale deeply, contracting abdomen.

6 Perform the identical slow, deep-controlled inhalation as in the standing position. During inhalation the shoulders, not arms, are slowly raised to extreme position. Palms remain on thighs.

Hold position and retain air for a count of 5.

Slowly exhale and simultaneously contract abdomen and lower shoulders to starting position of Fig. 5.

Without pause, repeat.

Perform 3 times during learning period.

Notes

Practice to gain control of the abdominal muscles so that you can contract and distend the abdomen as instructed.

The inhalations and exhalations must be executed slowly so that you can coordinate the slow raising and lowering of the arms and shoulders with your breathing.

All breathing is done quietly. Feel the breath more in the throat than in the nose.

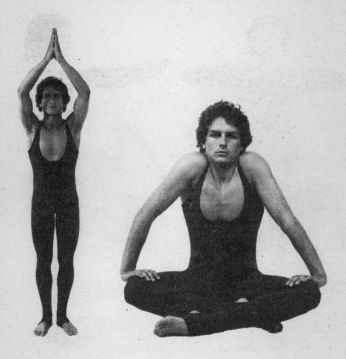

Do not:

bend the elbows, move arms forward, or permit the posture to become weak.

become tense in raising the shoulders or retaining the breath. Position is firm but relaxed. Spine remains straight.

(2) chest expansion

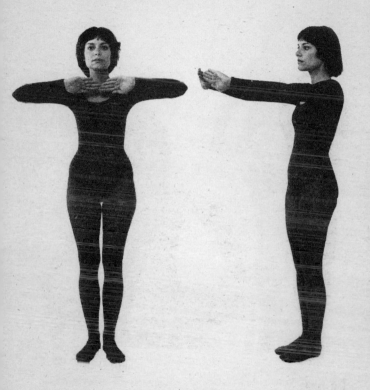

1 Stand erect with feet together and arms at sides.
  Slowly and gracefully raise arms into position illustrated, palms facing
    outward.
2 Slowly and gracefully extend arms straight outward at chest level.

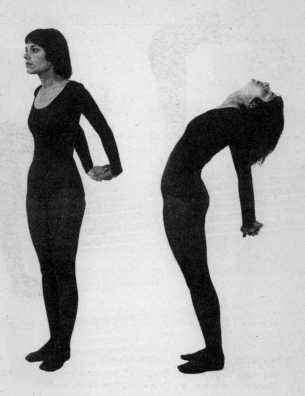

3 Slowly bring arms behind back and interlace fingers. Raise arms as high as possible while holding spine straight.

4 Bend very gently backward as far as possible **without strain.**
Knees are straight, head bent backward, neck relaxed, arms raised.
Hold without movement for a count of 5.

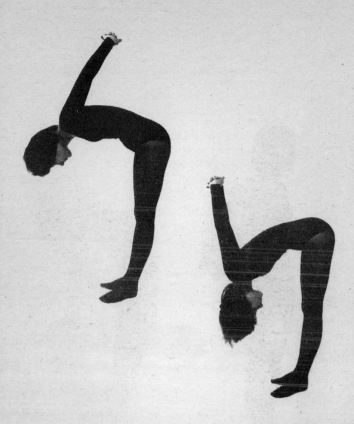

5 Very slowly straighten to the upright position.

Very slowly begin to bend forward. Fingers remain locked, arms come forward, knees straight, neck relaxed, and eyes open.

6 Continue to bend forward as far as possible without strain.

Hold without movement for a count of 10.

Very slowly straighten to the upright position.

Return arms to sides. Relax but remain still.

Perform twice during learning period.

Notes

You must never experience any strain in Yoga. Move very cautiously into the backward and forward bends. **Do not go farther than is comfortable.**

Keep the neck relaxed, eyes open, and arms high throughout the exercise.

Hold the backward and forward bends without movement for exactly the indicated count. It is the static **holds** that remove stiffness throughout the spine. A surprising degree of flexibility can be rapidly attained. With practice, your head may touch your knees. Breathe normally throughout this and the following *asanas*, unless otherwise instructed.

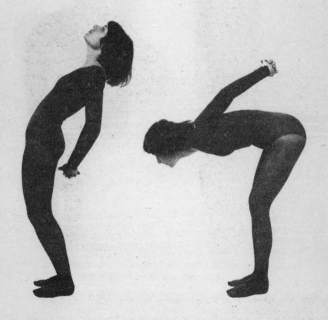

Do not:

bend knees or hold neck rigid. Notice how model has erroneously dropped arms in both positions.

(3) rishi's posture

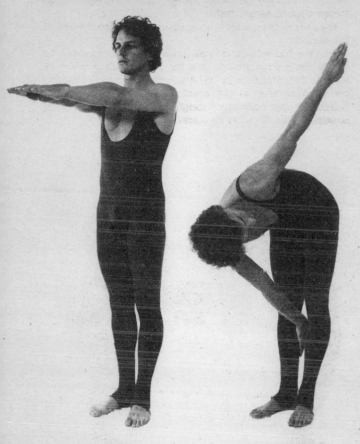

1 With feet slightly apart, raise arms as depicted. Palms face down.

2 Slowly bend forward at the waist and move right hand down along the inside **back** of the right leg. Knees are straight.

Simultaneously raise left arm (elbow straight) behind you. Turn head and twist trunk so that eyes see the **back** of the left hand.

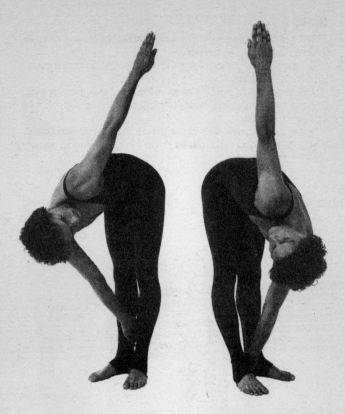

3 Continue to bend forward until right hand reaches furthermost part of right leg that it can hold without strain as eyes focus on back of left hand. Knees remain straight.

Hold without motion for 10.

Slowly straighten up, bringing arms into original outstretched position of Fig. 1.

4 Execute identical movements on opposite side. (More advanced position is depicted.)

Straighten to upright position of Fig. 1 and repeat.

Following final repetition, slowly lower arms to sides and relax.

During learning period, perform twice on each side, alternating sides.

Notes

Think of these movements as a slow-motion ballet and execute them as gracefully as possible.

Carefully note *right* and *left* in the directions to be sure that you hold the correct leg.

The hand should hold the **back** of the leg, not its front or side. Don't just touch the leg; **hold it firmly** and twist the trunk fully against this **hold.**

You must always be able to see the back of the upraised hand. If you cannot, you have raised it too high. The knees remain straight throughout.

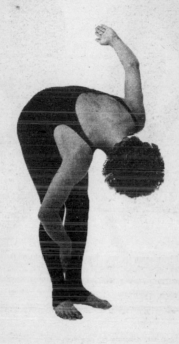

Do not:

bend knees or elbow of upraised arm. Model is touching side rather than firmly holding back of leg and is not twisting trunk and head sufficiently far to see back of hand.

(4) triangle

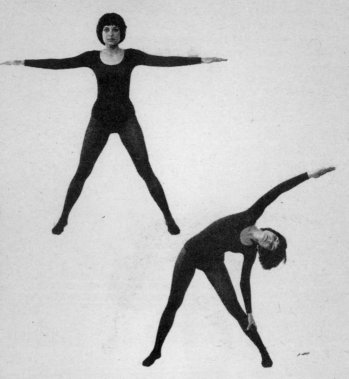

1 In a standing position, slowly separate legs and gracefully raise arms (palms down) as depicted.

2 Slowly bend to the left. Without strain, left hand holds lowermost outside area of left leg it can reach.

   Right arm, with elbow straight, comes over, stretching as far as possible.

   Knees straight; neck relaxed.

   Hold without movement for 10.

   Slowly straighten upright to position of Fig. 1. Arms are once again outstretched to the sides.

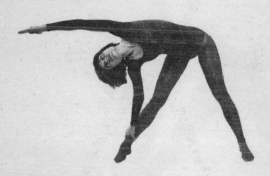

3 Execute identical movements to the right side.

(Note that photograph depicts model holding ankle rather than calf. The more extreme positions result from practice.)

Hold without movement for 10.

Slowly straighten to the upright position with arms outstretched. Repeat.

Following final repetition, slowly lower arms to sides and bring legs together. Relax.

During learning period, perform 3 times on each side, alternating sides.

Notes

Be sure to bring the arm as far over the head as possible. This aids in firming the sides. (Elbow must be straight and palm facing downward.)

Straighten to the upright position very slowly to help tone the muscles.

As you become proficient in this *asana* you can assume an increasingly wider stance to intensify the firming action.

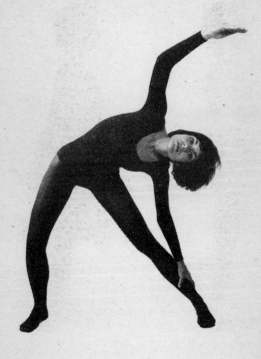

Do not:

bend elbow or hold neck rigid. Model is incorrectly bending right knee and has failed to bring arm over a sufficient distance to achieve the desired effect.

(5) balance posture

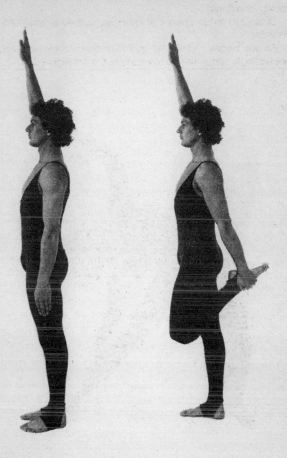

1 With heels together, slowly raise right arm to overhead position, fingers together.

2 Shift your weight onto the right leg. Bring left leg up so that left hand can hold left foot as depicted.

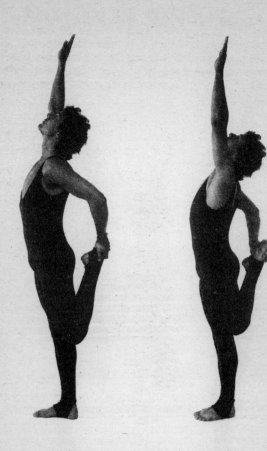

3 Pull up on left foot. Simultaneously look upward and move upraised
arm backward a few inches.

Hold as steady as possible for 5.

Slowly return arm to side and foot to floor.

4 Perform identical movements on opposite side.

During learning period, perform 3 times on each side, alternating
sides.

Notes

If you lose your balance at any point, pause a moment and begin again. Do not laugh at yourself. If you are unsuccessful in three attempts, proceed to the next technique. Repeated attempts over a period of time will bring success, and this success imparts balance, poise, and greater self-confidence. Balance is well worth cultivating, so be patient if your initial attempts do not meet with instant success.

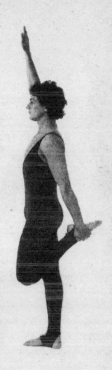

Do not:

neglect to stretch. Frequently, students are content to have accomplished the position depicted in Fig. 5 and fail to raise the foot or move the upraised arm to the overhead position. Be sure that the head tilts backward and the eyes look upward.

(6) dancer's movements

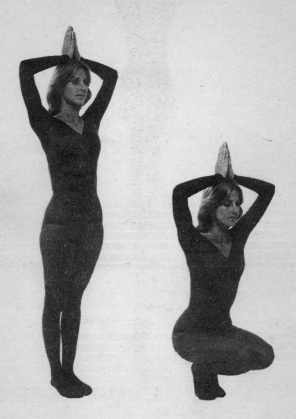

1 With heels together, rest hands on head as depicted. Palms are pressed together, fingers point straight upward.

2 In very slow motion, bend knees and lower trunk until buttocks touch heels. Knees remain together throughout movements.

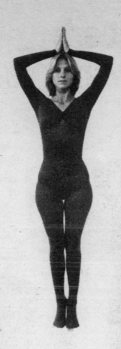

3 Without pause, very slowly raise body to the upright position and come up high on toes.

Hold as steady as possible for 5.

Slowly lower soles to floor and repeat.

Following final repetition, lower arms to sides and relax.

During learning period perform 5 times.

Notes

Very slow motion is essential to achieve the desired firming and strengthening of the legs.

Keep knees together. When buttocks touch heels, do not pause but immediately begin the upward movement.

If you lose your balance at any point, pause a moment and begin again. Do not laugh at yourself. Your body will respond to a serious mental approach.

(7) **back stretch**

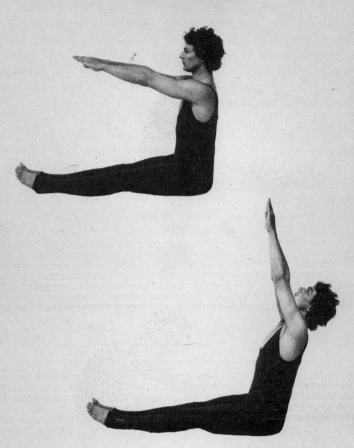

1 Seated on your mat with legs extended and together, slowly raise arms. Hands are close together.

2 Continue slow raising of arms to upward position. Bend trunk and head backward several inches and look upward.

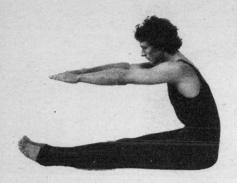

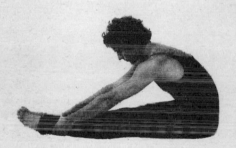

3 Execute a slow-motion dive forward.

4 Take a firm hold on the furthermost part of the legs that can be reached without strain.

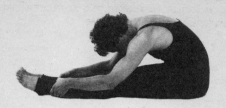

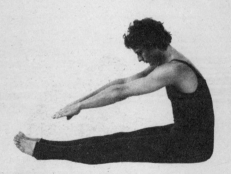

5 Lower forehead as far toward knees as possible without strain.

Knees straight, neck relaxed, elbows bent.

Hold without motion for 20.

6 Release legs and slowly straighten trunk to upright position; simultaneously raise arms as in Fig. 1.

Repeat

Following final repetition, rest hands on knees.

During learning period, perform 3 times.

Notes

Do not strain to go further than is comfortable. Even holding the knees is a satisfactory beginning position.

Bending the trunk backward (Fig. 2) helps to tone the abdominal muscles.

In Fig. 5, elbows must bend outward to help in lowering the trunk, and neck must be relaxed with forehead aimed toward knees to stretch the cervical vertebrae.

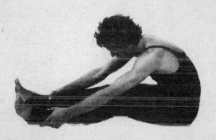

Do not:

separate legs, bend knees, hold elbows straight, or keep neck rigid and head raised.

(8) alternate leg stretch

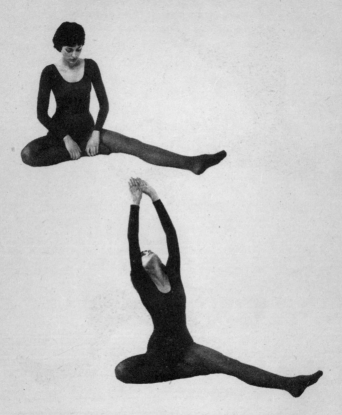

1 Legs are extended. Take right foot with hands and place it so that heel is as far in as possible and sole rests against inside of left thigh.

2 Slowly raise arms to overhead position. Bend trunk and head backward and look upward. Right knee must remain as close to floor as possible.

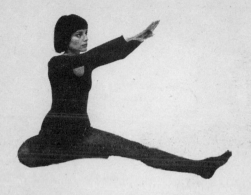

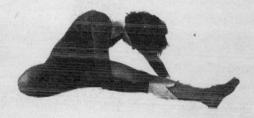

3 Execute a slow-motion dive, and with both hands firmly hold the furthermost part of the left leg that can be reached without strain.

4 Slowly and gently lower forehead as far toward left knee as possible.

Left knee straight, neck relaxed, elbows bent outward, right knee remains as close to floor as possible.

Hold without motion for 20.

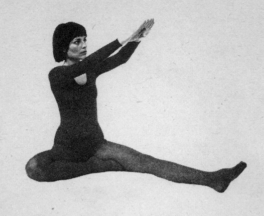

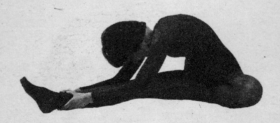

5 Release leg, slowly straighten trunk to upright position; simultaneously raise arms.

Repeat.

6 Execute identical movements with right leg extended. (More advanced position is depicted.)

Following final repetition, extend both legs and rest hands on knees.

During learning period, perform twice with left leg, then twice with right leg.

Notes

Be sure that the knee of the extended leg does not bend.

All Notes of previous posture, the Back Stretch, also apply here.

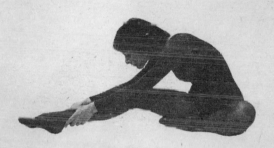

Do not:

bend knee of extended leg, allow knee of opposite leg to be raised higher than absolutely necessary, hold elbows straight or neck rigid. Model is simply touching calf and neglecting to take a firm hold.

(9) knee and thigh stretch

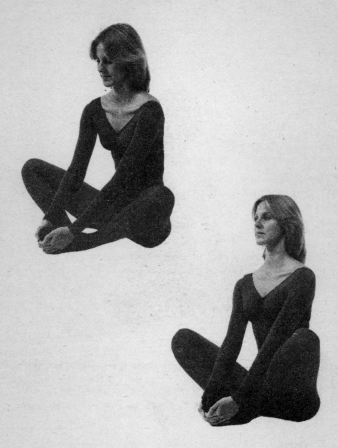

1 Clasp hands around feet and interlace fingers.

2 Bring feet in as far as possible. Straighten spine and head.

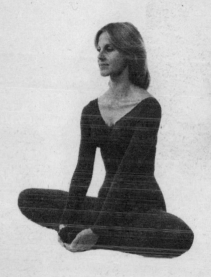

3 Pull up against feet to assist in slowly lowering knees as far as possible toward floor.

Hold without motion for 10.

Allow knees and thighs to relax for a few moments. Hands remain clasped around feet.

Repeat.

Following final repetition, release feet and slowly extend legs.

During learning period, perform 3 times.

Notes

Even if your knees can be lowered only several inches, this *asana* will be of value. As tightness in the thighs is worked out, knees can be lowered an increased distance.

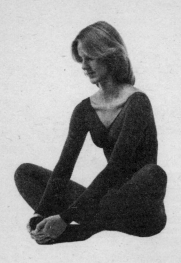

Do not:

allow the trunk to slump. Model has not drawn feet in as far as they will go, and she is not pulling up with sufficient strength to permit a lowering of the knees against this pull.

(10) **twist**

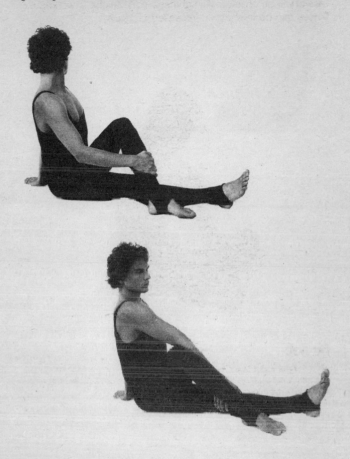

1 Legs are extended. Cross left leg over right and rest sole of foot on
   floor.
   Place left hand firmly on floor behind your back (for balance).

2 Cross right arm **over** left knee and take firm hold of right knee or calf
   with right hand.

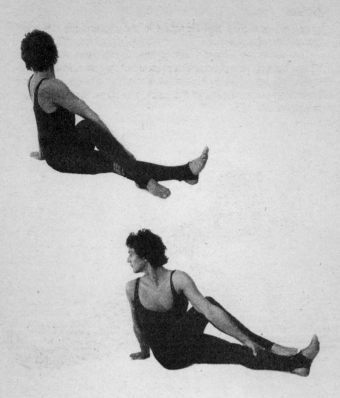

3 Very slowly turn head and twist trunk as far as possible to the **left.** Keep trunk erect.

Hold without motion for 10.

Slowly return head and trunk to the forward position of Fig. 2. Relax a few moments.

Repeat the twisting movement of Fig. 3.

4 Following the final repetition, extend legs and perform identical movements on opposite side. (Carefully exchange words *left* and *right* in the above directions.)

During learning period, perform 3 times on left side, then 3 times on right side.

Notes

At first, you may feel cramped in the movements. This will disappear with practice.

The vertebrae respond well to this "corkscrew" movement. Spinal twisting is a standard technique of the chiropractor. Students frequently feel exhilarated after this *asana* because there is an immediate loosening of the back and spine and a resultant freeing of energy.

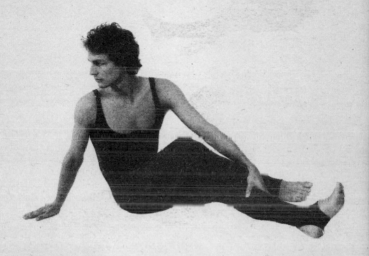

Do not:

allow trunk to slump or hand to reach **around** the knee rather than **over** it. Notice how the model does not have sole of foot on floor; hand is resting to the side of the back rather than behind it; trunk and head are not fully turned so that the full benefit of the corkscrew movement can be experienced.

(11) backward bend

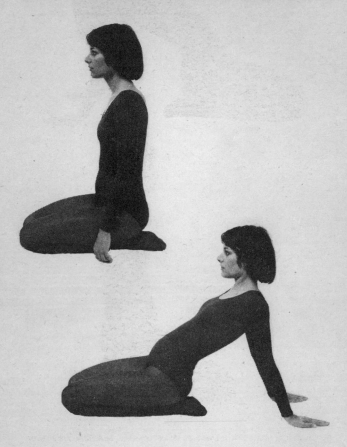

1 Sit on heels. Knees together, arms at sides.

2 Place palms on floor behind back and slowly inch backward a comfortable distance.

Knees together, arms even with sides, fingers together and pointing directly toward rear.

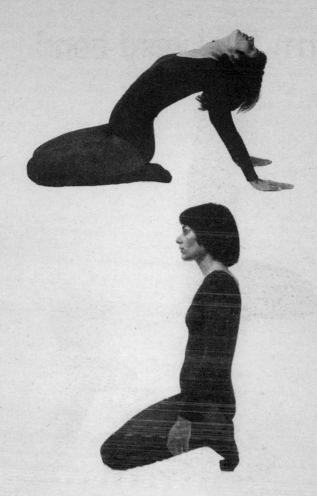

3 Cautiously arch trunk upward as far as possible; simultaneously lower head backward as far as possible. Do not raise buttocks from heels.

Hold without motion for 20.

Slowly raise head, lower trunk, inch hands forward to beginning position of Fig. 1.

4 Change position of feet so that toes are on floor.

Slowly lower buttocks to heels.

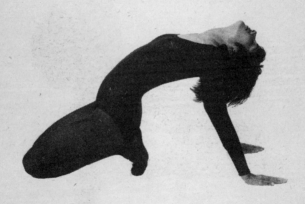

5 Place fingertips or palms on floor and cautiously inch backward a moderate distance.

Arch the spine and lower the head.

Hold without motion for 10.

Slowly raise head, lower trunk, inch hands forward to starting position of Fig. 4.

Bring legs out from beneath you and extend them straight outward.

During learning period, perform each of the 2 positions once.

Notes

Weakness and inflexibility are responsible for many negative conditions in the ankles, feet, and toes. The Backward Bend is one of several *asanas* that helps to prevent or relieve such conditions.

In executing the movements of Figs. 3 and 5, move very cautiously and stop whenever the position begins to become uncomfortable. Hold at that point for the indicated count, and within a few days you will be able to move further backward. **Never lunge forward or backward.**

The position depicted in Fig. 5 may be difficult. In the beginning you may not be able to go beyond simply sitting on your heels for a few moments. This is perfectly satisfactory. With continued practice, your toes will gain the necessary strength to support your weight and you can then proceed.

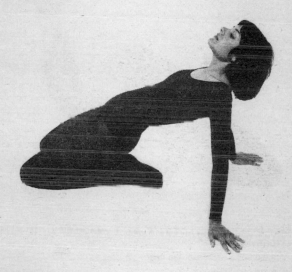

Do not:

separate knees, raise buttocks from heels, or neglect to lower head backward as far as possible. Notice how model's arms are not even with sides, fingers are not together and pointing directly to rear, and spine is not fully arched.

(12) **shoulder stand**

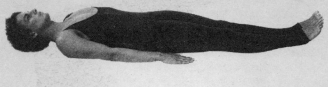

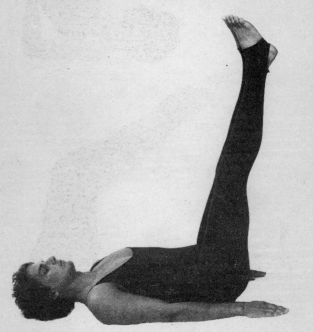

1 Lie on back, arms at sides, palms on floor.

2 Stiffen leg and abdominal muscles. Push against floor with hands and slowly raise legs (knees straight).

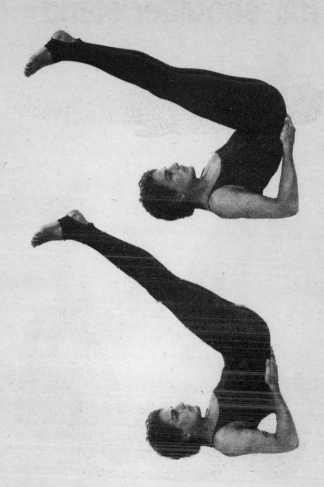

3 Swing legs back over head.
  Place hands firmly against lower back or hips.

4 Slowly straighten legs and trunk.
  Stop at that point where straightening begins to become uncomfortable.

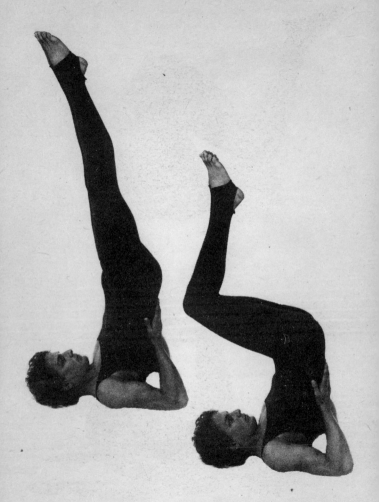

5 The completed position (accomplished with patient practice).
Hold your extreme position without motion for 30–60 seconds during
learning period.

6 Bend knees and slowly lower them toward head.

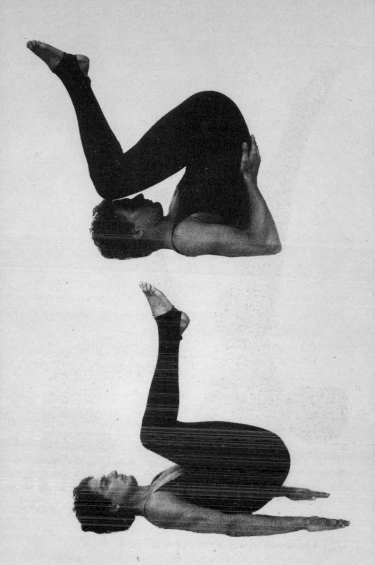

7 Continue to lower knees as far as possible.

8 Place hands on floor and **slowly** roll forward.

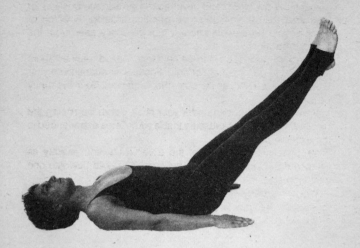

9 When lower back touches floor, extend legs straight outward and very slowly lower them to floor.

10 Allow body to relax completely for approximately 1 minute. (See Fig. 1.)

The Shoulder Stand is performed only once.

Notes

Any angle of inversion is of value, so even if you are able to attain only a very modified position of the Shoulder Stand you will benefit accordingly, and you will gradually be able to straighten to the more advanced position. There need be no hurry to attain the completed posture. Take as much time as is necessary to become comfortable in each of the preceding positions.

Swinging the legs back over the head (Fig. 3) assists in raising the lower back from the floor. If necessary, this movement can be done more quickly to gain momentum.

Begin the hold in your extreme position with 30–60 seconds. The **Fitness Programs** and **Special Routines** require the extreme position to be held for longer periods. These more extended periods are accomplished by adding 15 seconds each week until the indicated time is reached. Do not add more than 15 seconds per week, and never hold your extreme position for **less** time than in your previous practice session. A watch or clock should be placed where it can be easily seen from the inverted position.

The extreme position is to be held in a relaxed manner. There is no need to become tight or rigid. Focus your attention on your breathing which should be slow and controlled. Your eyes may be closed.

A folded towel placed under your neck before beginning the movements will relieve pressure that is sometimes experienced in the extreme position.

Be certain to come out of the extreme position **exactly** as instructed in Figs. 6–9. These movements should flow into one another, being smooth and continuous.

When you have returned to the horizontal position and allowed the body to become limp, you will experience a deep relaxation and a subsequent rovitalization

(13) plough

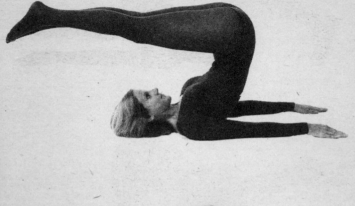

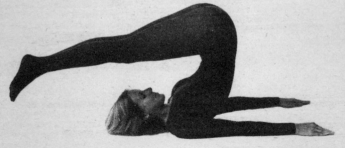

1 Lie on back. Proceed exactly as in the Shoulder Stand (12), and bring legs back over head.

2 Instead of straightening trunk as in the Shoulder Stand, keep palms on floor and continue to bring legs back.

Slowly lower legs as far as possible toward floor. Stop at that point where lowering of legs begins to become uncomfortable.

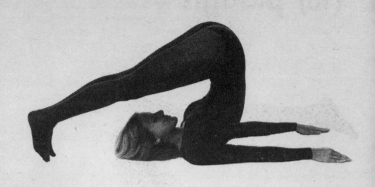

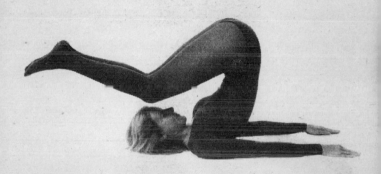

3 In final position (gradually attained with practice), feet touch floor **as close to head as possible.**

In Figs. 2 and 3 legs remain together and knees are straight.

Hold your extreme position for 20.

4 Bend knees and bring them toward forehead.

Proceed from this point exactly as in the Shoulder Stand until entire body rests on floor.

Relax for approximately 30 seconds.

Repeat.

During learning period perform twice.

Notes

The final position depicted in Fig. 3 is accomplished with patient practice. If you will simply hold **your** extreme position, regardless of how far your feet are from the floor, the weight of your legs will enable you to gain the necessary flexibility. There is no value in forcing the legs to a position that is lower than comfortable. Any straining will only retard your progress. Always remember that all of the benefits you will derive from Yoga practice are gained through the holding of **your** extreme positions.

In the first few attempts, your breathing may be irregular because of the way your chin is pressed against your chest, but if you concentrate on the breathing you will soon be able to normalize it.

By performing the Plough very slowly, you are able to emphasize each vertebra in turn, thus manipulating the entire back and spine.

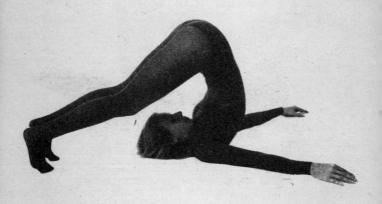

Do not:

bend knees, move arms away from sides, raise palms from floor, or separate legs and feet.

(14) **cobra**

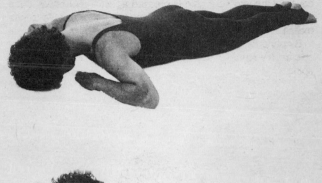

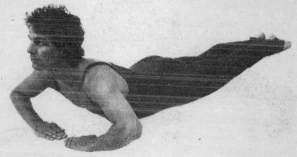

1 Rest forehead on mat. Place hands beneath shoulders; fingers are together and point toward opposite hand. (The correct hand and finger position is very important.)

2 Slowly raise head.
Tilt head backward and begin to very slowly raise trunk by pushing hands against floor.

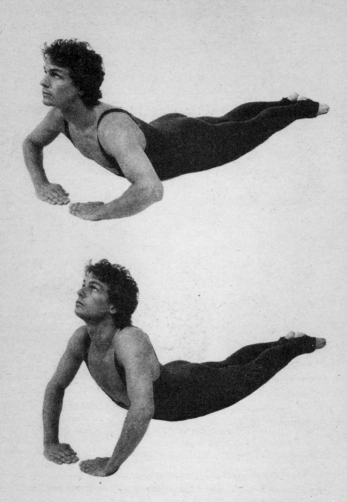

3 Continue to very slowly raise trunk. Spine must be curved throughout movements and head tilted backward.

4 Raise as high as is comfortable.

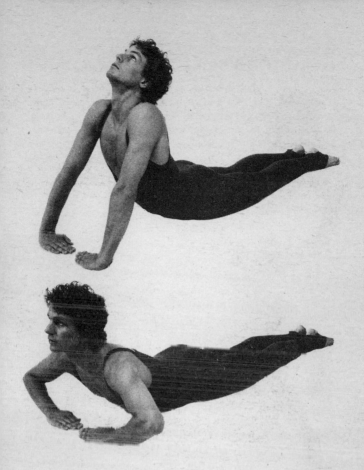

5 In extreme position elbows are straight, head back, lower abdomen touching floor, and legs relaxed.

Hold your extreme position without motion for 15.

6 Reverse the movements and very slowly lower trunk to floor.

Return arms to sides, rest cheek on mat, and relax completely for approximately 30 seconds.

Repeat.

During learning period perform 3 times.

Notes

Your head must be continually tilted backward with eyes looking upward. Spine is continually arched, never straightened.

Be sure that the hand and finger positions are correct. (Hands beneath shoulders, fingers point inward toward opposite hand. This hand position enables you to raise the trunk the correct distance in the final position.)

Raise your trunk only as high as is comfortable. Hold this position without motion for 15. You will probably find yourself raising an inch higher in each practice session.

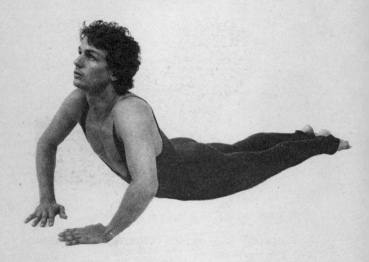

Do not:

tense legs or spread fingers and point them away from trunk. Notice how by neglecting to tilt head backward, model has lost cervical and dorsal curvature.

(15) **neck movements**

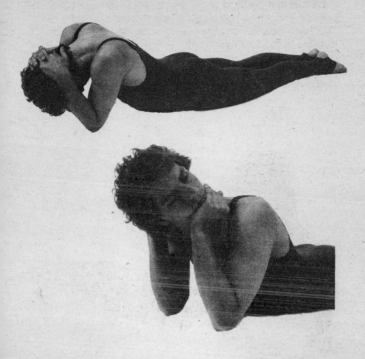

1 Lying on abdomen, place elbows on floor, approximately 9 inches
apart. Arms are parallel.

Clasp hands on back of head—just above neck—and gently push
head down as far as possible. (Eventually, chin should press against
top of chest.)

Hold without motion for 10.

2 Slowly raise head and rest chin in left palm with fingers together on left
cheek. Place right hand firmly on back of head.

Use hands to slowly turn head as far as possible to left. (Elbows remain
on floor.)

Hold without motion for 10.

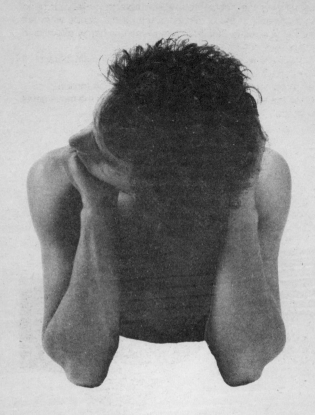

3 Do not move arms. Turn head and rest chin in right palm; left hand
grips back of head.

Use hands to slowly turn head as far as possible to right.

Hold without motion for 10.

Turn head to front position.

Repeat.

Following final repetition, lower chin to mat and return arms to sides.

During learning period perform the 3 movements twice.

Notes

By utilizing the hands, you will be able to move your head further in each of the 3 directions than if the hands were not assisting. This extra half-inch of movement is highly effective in reaching the stiff, tense areas.

Elbows are on the floor throughout; arms remain parallel. If elbows spread, you will not have sufficient height.

All movements must be executed in very slow motion.

Once learned, the eyes may be closed during the movements and **holds.**

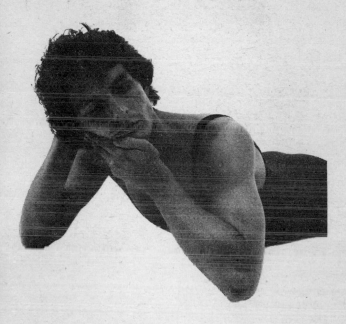

Do not:

spread elbows farther than directed. Notice how model has fingers on the incorrect cheek. In turning to the left (Fig. 2) fingers are on the left cheek; in turning to the right, fingers are on the right cheek. Model is simply resting head in hands rather than having hands firmly grip the back of the head, cheek, and chin.

(16) locust

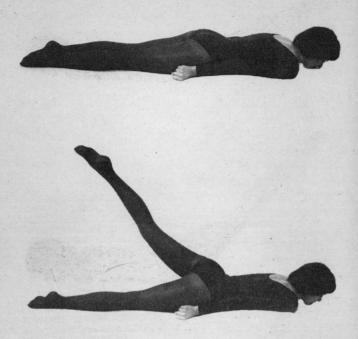

1 Rest chin on mat. Make fists and place them at sides, thumbs down.

2 Push down with fists and slowly raise left leg as high as possible. Chin
  remains on floor.

  Hold without motion for 10.

  Slowly lower left leg to floor.

  Execute identical movements with right leg, holding your extreme
  position for 10.

  Perform 3 times with each leg, alternating from left to right.

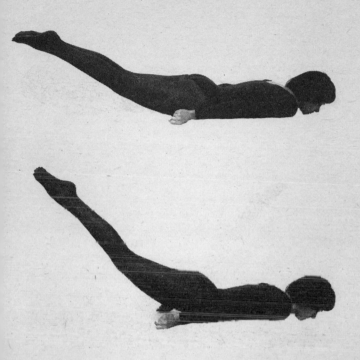

3 Inhale deeply and slowly through nose and retain breath.

Push fists hard against floor and raise both legs as high as possible without strain.

Legs are together, knees straight. Chin must not leave floor.

Hold with as little motion as possible for 5.

Slowly lower legs to floor; simultaneously slowly exhale.

Relax a few moments and repeat.

4 A more advanced position that is accomplished with patient practice.

During learning period, perform the position with both legs, twice.

71

Notes

The benefits of the Locust are gained by performing the movements to the best of your ability, not by how high your legs are raised. As muscle tone is acquired in the arms, abdomen, and legs, the height of the raise will increase.

For better support, rest your head more toward the mouth than the point of the chin.

The inhalation and retention of breath (Fig. 3) enlarges the chest for better support during raising of the legs. Keeping the legs together during the raise places additional emphasis on the abdomen and buttocks.

The lowering of both legs must be done with control. Do not "collapse" and permit your legs to fall to the floor; lower them slowly. The exhalation should be through the nose, slow and quiet. Do not allow the breath to gush out.

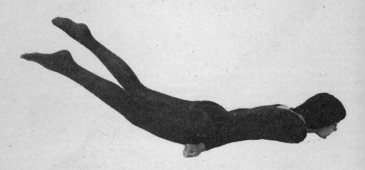

Do not:

bend knees, spread legs, or position arms away from sides. Notice how model has placed **point** of chin on floor; she is incorrectly resting all fingers of fists on floor rather than turning the fists on their sides so that only the thumbs and index fingers touch floor.

(17) **bow**

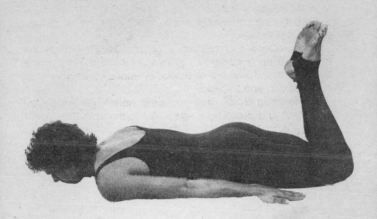

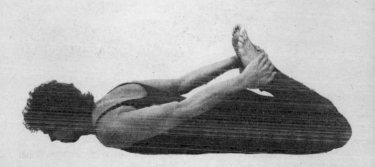

1 Rest chin on mat, arms at sides.
Bend knees and bring feet toward back.

2 Reach back and hold feet firmly.

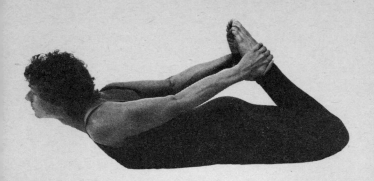

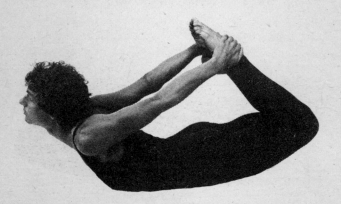

3 Pull against feet and cautiously, slowly, and gently raise trunk. Head is tilted backward.

4 Continue to pull against feet and raise knees and thighs.

Trunk and legs are now raised as high as possible without strain.

Knees are close together; head is back.

Hold without motion for 10.

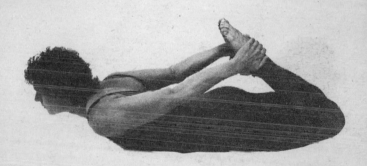

5 To come out of position, lower knees to floor **first;** then lower chin to floor but maintain hold on feet.

Rest several moments. Repeat.

Following final repetition, return knees and chin to floor; release feet and lower them slowly to floor. Rest cheek on floor and relax completely.

Perform 3 times during learning period.

Notes

At first you may have to struggle to hold both feet. Continued attempts will bring success. In your initial practice sessions you can hold one foot and then let go and try to hold the other. This practice will soon enable you to hold both feet.

Raising the trunk (Fig. 3) is not difficult, but raising the knees and thighs (Fig. 4) usually requires practice to develop the necessary muscle action.

Keeping the knees together during the raise places added emphasis on the spine. Holding the head back during the raise aids in the spinal curvature.

In lowering (Fig. 5) be sure that the chin is brought to the floor **first** and **then** lower the knees to the floor.

Proceed very cautiously and never make any sudden or erratic movement. Practice to achieve slowness and control.

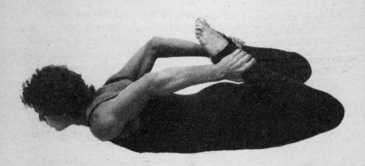

Do not:

separate knees, hold ankles rather than feet, or neglect to bend head backward. Because model is not pulling with sufficient strength on feet, he is unable to raise the trunk.

the *complete* daily fitness program

This **Complete** plan comprises two routines (AM and PM) that incorporate the Seventeen Basic Techniques. The **AM Routine** is for morning practice, ideally before breakfast, but any time of the morning is satisfactory. In the early morning the body is relatively "stiff" from the night's sleep and you should not be concerned about how well you accomplish extreme positions at that time. Actually, the *asanas* will work out stiffness and tension accumulated during the night, free trapped energy, and prepare you physically and mentally for the day's activities. If early morning practice is impractical, aim for a midmorning session. The earlier in the day that you can perform the **AM Routine,** the better.

The **PM Routine** is for afternoon or evening practice. It is an excellent routine to perform when returning home from the day's work (prior to dinner). However exhausted you may feel at that hour, if you perform the **PM Routine** before resting or eating you will find yourself wonderfully refreshed and invigorated within the hour. For those who work at home, the middle or late afternoon is an advantageous time for this routine. Because of its revitalizing effects, the **PM Routine** is not suggested immediately prior to retiring for the night. (There is a **Special Routine** to help induce restful sleep.)

Once the *asanas* have been learned, each of the two routines can be leisurely performed in thirty minutes. It is recommended that you practice at approximately the same AM and PM hours each day. The routines are in standing, sitting, and lying sequence. The following pages depict two positions of each *asana* in the routines, so that once learned, a glance at the photographs will remind you of the movements. However, be sure to refer to the appropriate directions, photographs, and notes of the first section until each *asana* is thoroughly learned. (If, subsequently, you elect to learn the advanced positions, you will include these in your practice. You may also wish to include one or more of the **Special Routines** with the **Fitness Program.** Information regarding these possibilities is presented in the pertinent sections.) Carefully note the number of repetitions that is indicated for each *asana* of these routines because it is not necessarily the same as that for the "learning period" in the Basic Techniques.

Each routine concludes with a Continuous Motion performance of the *asanas*. This means that you perform all of the *asanas* in the routine in consecutive order, once each, without holding the extreme position and without pause between the *asanas*. The entire routine becomes a continuous slow-motion dance without any pause.

Always remember the cumulative value of **daily practice.** When your practice hour arrives, do not allow your mind to put you off with the many "more important" matters it will invent, and which it will insist must absolutely be attended to at that moment. If you can disregard these distractions and persevere with daily sessions for two months, the results will be so gratifying that, thereafter, your body will seldom permit you to skip a day of practice.

complete fitness program— am routine

complete breath standing (1A)

Perform 5 times. Retain each breath for a count of 5.

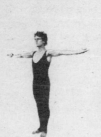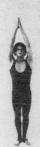

chest expansion (2)

Perform twice. Hold the backward bends for 5 and the forward bends for 10.

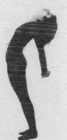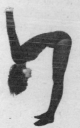

triangle (4)

Perform 3 times on each side, alternating from left to right. Hold each stretch for 10.

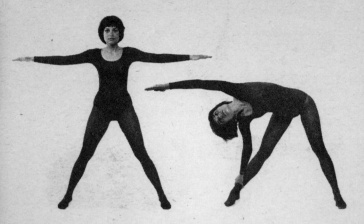

dancer's movements (6)

Perform 5 times. Hold the toes position for 5.

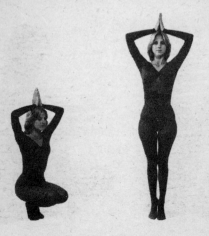

back stretch (7)

Perform twice. Hold each stretch for 20.

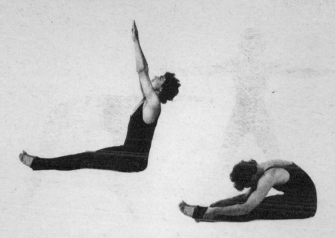

knee and thigh stretch (9)

Perform 3 times. Hold each stretch for 10.

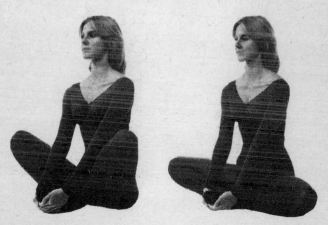

twist (10)

Perform 3 times on left side, then 3 times on right side. Hold each twist for 10.

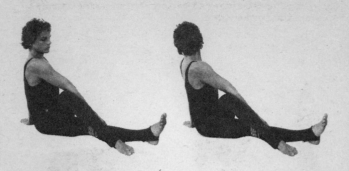

backward bend (11)

Perform each of the 2 positions once. Hold each stretch for 20.

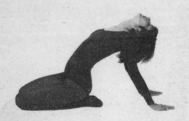

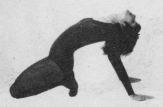

continuous motion

Begin with the Complete Breath Standing (1A) and perform each of the *asanas*, in consecutive order, once. There is no holding of the extreme positions and no pause between the *asanas*. The entire routine becomes a continuous slow-motion dance.

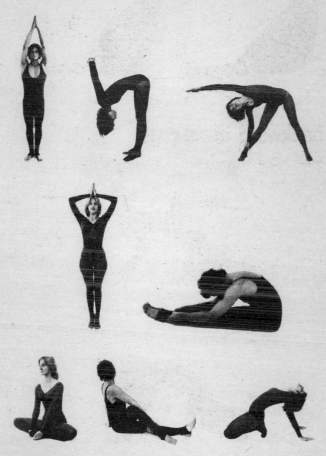

Upon completion of Continuous Motion, conclude the session with the following technique:

complete breath seated (1B)

Perform 5 times. Retain each breath for 5.

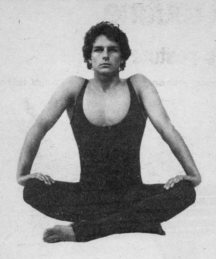

complete fitness program— pm routine

rishi's posture (3)

Perform twice on each side, alternating from left to right. Hold each stretch for 10.

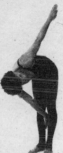 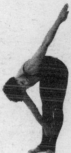

balance posture (5)

Perform 3 times on each side, alternating sides. Hold each stretch for 5.

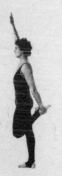 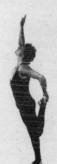

alternate leg stretch (8)

Perform twice with left leg, then twice with right leg. Hold each stretch for 20.

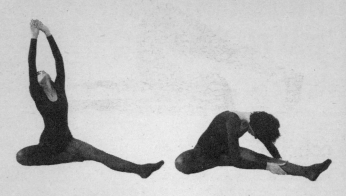

shoulder stand (12)

Perform once. Hold 3–5 minutes.

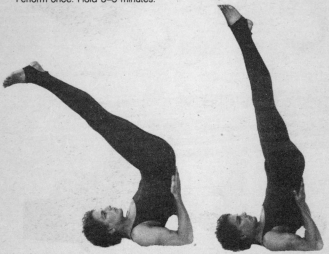

plough (13)

Perform twice. Hold each for 20

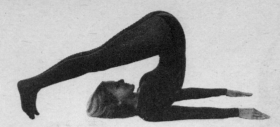

cobra (14)

Perform 3 times. Hold each raise for 20.

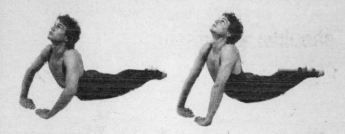

neck movements (15)

Perform the 3 movements twice. Hold each position for 10.

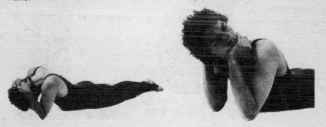

locust (16)

Perform twice. Hold each raise for 5–10.

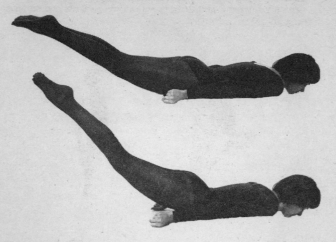

bow (17)

Perform twice. Hold each raise for 10–20.

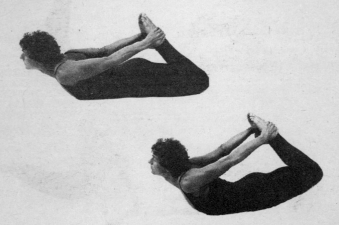

continuous motion

Begin with Rishi's Posture and perform each of the *asanas*, in consecutive order, once. There is no holding of the extreme positions and no pause between *asanas*.

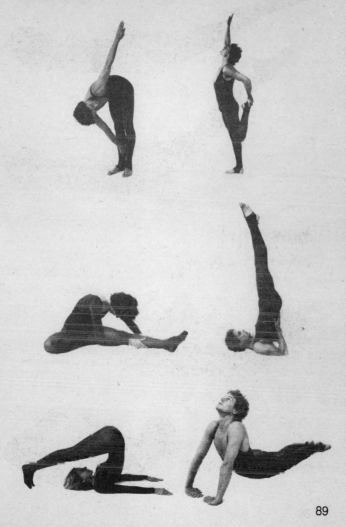

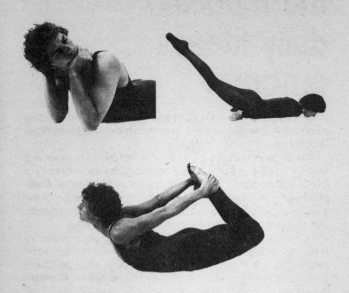

Upon completion of Continuous Motion, conclude the session with the following technique:

complete breath seated (1B)

Perform 5 times. Retain each breath for 5. (This is the final technique of each routine. It induces a serene but aware state of consciousness.)

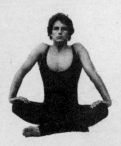

the *modified* daily fitness program

The **Modified** plan comprises two routines (AM and PM) that incorporate a selection of the *asanas* from the Seventeen Basic Techniques.

This program contains approximately half the techniques and requires half the practice time (fifteen minutes each routine) of the **Complete** plan. Therefore, it is less intensive than the **Complete** plan but still provides a satisfactory manipulation of the body and can serve as an excellent basis for maintaining health and fitness for those who are extremely limited in time.

Those who adopt this **Modified** plan for daily practice should attempt to also perform the **Complete** plan once or twice each week—during the weekends— or on those days when additional time is available. This extra practice will round out the **Modified Program.**

With the exception of the necessary practice time and the number of *asanas* that comprise the routines, all information presented on page 77 applies to this **Modified** plan. Refer to this information before proceeding.

modified fitness program— am routine

complete breath standing (1A)

Perform 5 times. Retain each breath for a count of 5.

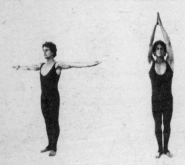

triangle (4)

Perform 3 times on each side, alternating from left to right. Hold each stretch for 10.

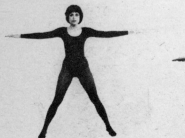
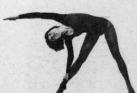

twist (10)

Perform 3 times on left side, then 3 times on right side. Hold each twist for 10.

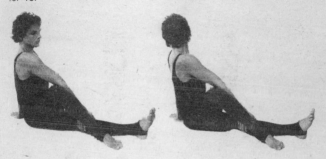

knee and thigh stretch (9)

Perform 3 times. Hold each stretch for 10.

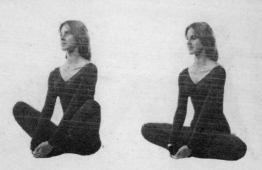

back stretch (7)

Perform twice. Hold each stretch for 20.

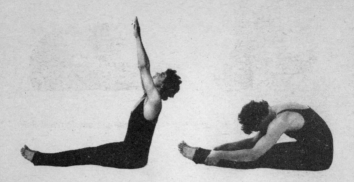

continuous motion

Begin with the Complete Breath Standing (1A) and perform each of the *asanas*, in consecutive order, once. There is no holding of the extreme positions and no pause between the *asanas*. The entire routine becomes a continuous slow-motion dance.

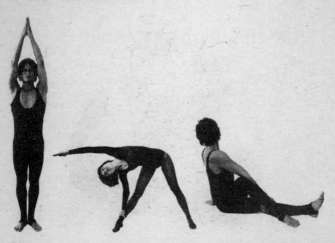

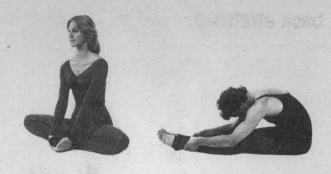

Upon completion of Continuous Motion, conclude the session with the following technique:

complete breath seated (1B)

Perform 5 times. Retain each breath for 5. (This is the final technique of each routine. It induces a serene but aware state of consciousness.)

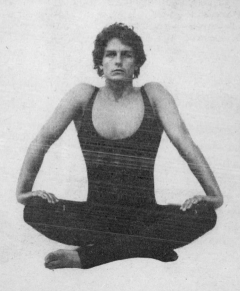

modified fitness program— pm routine

rishi's posture (3)

Perform twice on each side, alternating from left to right. Hold each stretch for 10.

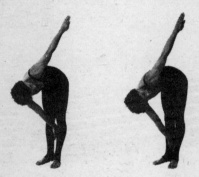

cobra (14)

Perform 3 times. Hold each raise for 20.

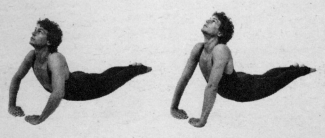

bow (17)

Perform twice. Hold each raise for 10–20.

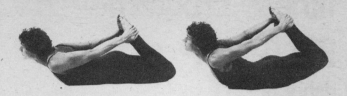

alternate leg stretch (8)

Perform twice with left leg, then twice with right leg. Hold each stretch for 20.

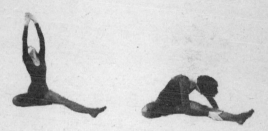

shoulder stand (12)

Perform once. Hold 3 minutes.

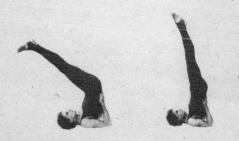

continuous motion

Begin with Rishi's Posture and perform each of the *asanas*, in consecutive order, once. There is no holding of the extreme positions and no pause between *asanas*.

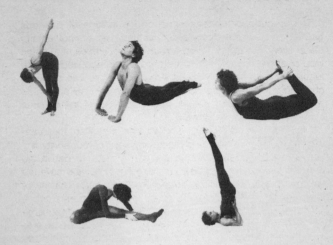

Upon completion of Continuous Motion, conclude the session with the following technique:

complete breath seated (1B)

Perform 5 times. Retain each breath for 5.

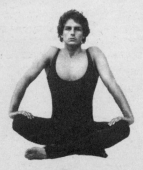

advanced techniques

This section comprises advanced positions of previous *asanas* and several classical techniques that are not among those already learned. These advanced techniques require the type of strength, control, and balance that is acquired through regular practice of the **Fitness Programs.** They can serve as challenges for future practice and can be cautiously attempted **once you feel totally secure in the *asanas* of the Fitness Program you have selected.**

Depending upon your age and physical condition, these advanced techniques may be permanently beyond your ability. It is not essential that you undertake them in order to derive the benefits previously listed. But for those students who have the capacity to make additional demands on their bodies, mastery of these advanced positions will offer increased benefits and a sense of accomplishment. It should also be noted that some students prematurely conclude that they will never be able to perform the advanced positions. These students do not understand the way in which Hatha Yoga works, and many are most pleasantly surprised when, after several months of serious practice, they have developed the ability to move into the advanced positions. The point is that no judgment should be made as to what your degree of proficiency may be several months from the time you begin the **Fitness Program.**

The manner in which the advanced work can be incorporated into the **Fitness Programs** and **Special Routines** is explained at the appropriate points. But remember that you must be in no hurry to attempt these positions. If you are not entirely comfortable in the Basic Techniques, you will not benefit from the advanced work and might even retard your progress. It is perfectly acceptable that you spend six months or longer in perfecting the basic *asanas*.

(18) abdominal lift

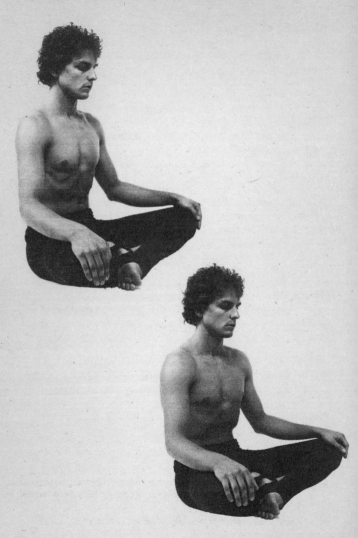

1 Sit in a simple cross-legged posture and rest your hands on your knees.

2 Fix your attention on the abdominal muscles. Contract these muscles as much as possible and attempt to create a fairly deep "hollow" in the abdominal area.

Hold whatever contraction you attain for a count of 3.

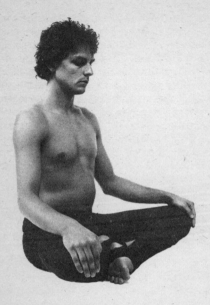

3 Use the same muscles to forcefully and quickly push the abdomen out (distend) as far as possible. (This is not simply a relaxing of the abdomen. It is a forceful, sudden distension or "snapping" out of the abdomen.)

Without pause repeat these contracting-distending movements with a hold of 3 seconds, 10 times. Upon completion, relax a few moments.

Perform the series of 10 movements 3 times, making a total of 30.

The above movements are practiced to prepare for the actual "lift" that follows. It is necessary that you strengthen these abdominal muscles and gain control of the contraction-distension movements to accomplish the lift. Once you have acquired this control you can proceed to the next step.

Notes

It is necessary to become proficient in the movements of Figs. 2 and 3 before proceeding to the complete lift. You may require a number of practice sessions to develop this proficiency. Actually, your practice of the preliminary movements will be as beneficial as the ultimate lift, especially if your abdominal muscles are weak or if you have become flabby in that area.

Some students learn the lift technique quickly; others require several weeks or longer. There is no hurry. With regular practice, the moment arrives when you suddenly get the knack of the lift, as you might get the knack of maintaining your balance on a bicycle. Therefore, do not become discouraged if your efforts do not meet with immediate success, and keep in mind that you will be continually benefiting from each practice session regardless of the depth of your contraction or lift.

Once you have perfected the lift, or feel that you have made good progress in the contractions, the exercise should be performed in the standing position that follows. This places the organs and glands in an advantageous position for stimulation.

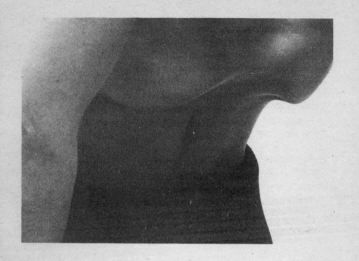

4 Study the photograph. Note that now the abdomen is not just contracted but **raised.** This raise requires control of the muscles and the emptying of the lungs through a deep and complete **exhalation** before the lift is attempted.

Exhale deeply and **keep all air out of the lungs.** This exhalation creates the vacuum that is necessary.

Imagine that you are going to take a deep breath from the pit of your stomach: use your abdominal muscles as you would your lungs, so that the abdomen is "sucked" inward and upward. (No air actually enters the lungs; this is a deep "breath" with the abdominal muscles, not the lungs.)

Hold the lift for 1 or 2 seconds and then quickly and forcefully "snap" the abdomen out as in Fig. 3.

Without pause and **without inhalation** perform 5 lifts. Then breathe normally and relax a few moments.

Execute the next deep exhalation and repeat the series of 5 lifts. Perform 5 series so that you do 25 lifts during the learning period.

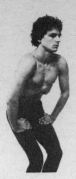

5 Study the photograph. In a standing position with your feet slightly apart, imagine that you are going to squat onto your heels, but go down only a few inches and stop.

Knees are bent slightly outward, hands are pressed firmly against upper thighs. Fingers (including thumbs) are together and turned inward.

Exhale deeply and perform the 5 lifts (or deep contractions).

Breathe normally, straighten upright, and pause a few moments but do not fidget.

Resume the position, exhale deeply, and repeat. Perform 5 rounds.

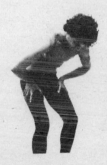

Do not:

hook thumb onto thigh, spread fingers or turn them outward, bend trunk forward rather than holding it straight and lowering it several inches. Notice how model has the legs too far apart and is bending head down.

Additional Notes

The key to success in these movements is cultivating the ability to empty the lungs completely in the exhalation and allow no air whatsoever to enter while the abdominal muscles perform the lift. If the lungs are even slightly expanded, you cannot properly execute the complete lift.

Remember that the movements do not constitute a continual **rolling** of the abdomen: there must be the brief **hold** of 3 seconds for the lift or deep contraction. Then the abdomen is not merely relaxed but "snapped" outward. Practice to make these movements crisp and rhythmic.

During the learning period it is suggested that you perform 5 rounds in each of the 2 positions (sitting and standing), making a total of 50 lifts. However, as your proficiency increases, it will become possible to execute 10 and more lifts to each exhalation. At that point you can perform approximately 100 lifts (10 lifts x 5 rounds x 2 positions) during the practice session.

If you wish to add this highly therapeutic technique to your daily **Fitness Program,** you should include it as the last standing technique of the **PM Routine.** This means that it would follow the Balance Posture (5) of the **Complete Program,** and Rishi's Posture (3) of the **Modified Program.**

(19) head stand

Place a small pillow or folded towel on your mat. This will serve to relieve pressure on the head and neck. Eventually, you may find that you do not require it, but it is a good idea to use it in the beginning stages. (In photographs, model is shown without pillow for clearer view of hands and head.) Position your watch or clock where you will be able to see it with your body in the inverted position. (Timepiece is not shown in photographs.)

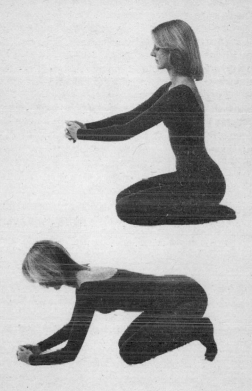

1 Kneeling on your mat, extend arms and interlace fingers.

2 Bend forward and place hands on pillow (or towel). Hands rest on their sides with thumbs facing up. Place toes on floor as illustrated.

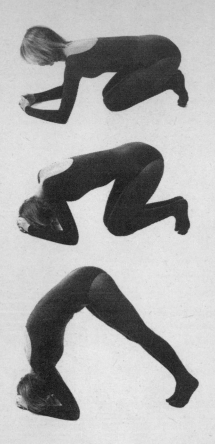

3 Lower elbows and forearms to floor. Clasped hands are now the apex of a triangle, with the forearms as the sides.

4 Lower head so that the top rests on the floor (pillow, or towel), and the back of the head is firmly cradled in clasped hands. (Be sure that the head is not resting on **top** of the hands. The hands are firmly holding the **back** of the head.)

5 Push down with your toes and forearms, and slowly raise the body into this arch.

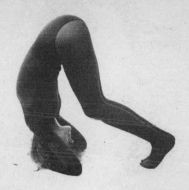

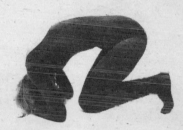

6 Inch toes slowly forward until knees are as close to chest as possible.

Do not straighten knees

Do not go beyond this position during first 10 practice sessions. (Keep a record.)

Hold as steady as possible for 30–60 seconds.

7 Slowly lower knees to floor. Very slowly raise head and come into a seated position.

This preparatory posture is performed once.

Beginning with the 11th practice session of the Head Stand:

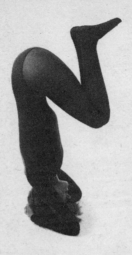

8 Proceeding from Fig. 6, shift full weight to head and forearms. Move trunk slightly forward and very slowly raise legs to illustrated position.

Feet and knees remain together. Back is straight.

Hold as steady as possible for 30–60 seconds.

If you lose your balance or are unable to attain the position, make another attempt. Three such attempts in a practice session are sufficient. If you are unsuccessful, terminate the posture and go on to the next technique.

You must be totally secure in this Modified Head Stand for 10 practice sessions before proceeding to the next stages. (Keep a record.)

Lower knees to floor and rest with head down for 30–60 seconds.

Slowly raise head and come into a seated position.

When you are totally secure in the position of Fig. 8:

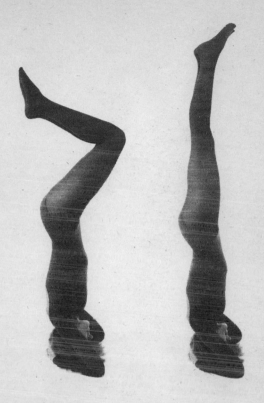

9 Very slowly and cautiously extend legs upward.

Legs must not be **thrust** upward. Legs remain together, back straight.

10 The completed Head Stand.

Hold as steady as possible. Any number of seconds is satisfactory; 30–60 seconds would be excellent for the first several weeks of the completed position. Gradually, additional seconds can be added—approximately 5 per week—until a maximum hold of 3 minutes is reached.

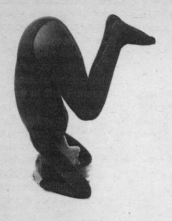

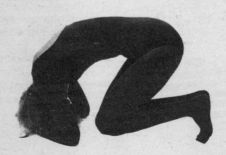

11 Very slowly bend knees and lower them to chest.

12 Slowly lower toes to floor. Then rest knees on floor and remain with head down for 30–60 seconds.

Slowly raise head and come into a seated position.

Notes

Tens of thousands of students who were at first extremely reluctant to even attempt the Head Stand have eventually accomplished the completed posture! I attribute this success to the fact that we make no attempt to spring into a full Head Stand like an expert gymnast; rather, we proceed with extreme caution and invert the body very gradually in a series of stages, feeling fully supported and in complete control each step of the way. We also stress that attaining the **complete** inversion need not necessarily be our objective because important benefits are derived from the modified positions.

While the Shoulder Stand locks the chin against the chest, directing the increased blood flow into the thyroid gland, the Head Stand directs the blood directly into the head. Nothing else can so quickly refresh the brain and aid in clarity of mind; you feel remarkably invigorated after a short period of time in this inverted position. Serious Yogis perform the Head Stand to also help awaken brain power that lies dormant. For many centuries, Yogis have maintained that most humans utilize only a fraction of what is a great untapped potential of energy and intelligence. The Head Stand is one of the *asanas* practiced to gain access to this potential

In Fig. 6, the closer you can bring your knees to your chest, the easier it will be to shift your weight to the head and forearms.

When you first invert the body you may experience some discomfort as the blood flows more fully into your head. This feeling of increased pressure usually disappears within one to two weeks of practice.

Carefully note the word *slowly* as it appears in the directions. If you catch yourself beginning to move too quickly, change that movement into slow motion. If you do not practice the completed position in slow motion, you will never be truly secure in the movements.

Never jump up suddenly when you have completed the posture. A sudden change can make you dizzy. Always rest with the head down, as indicated. Persons with high blood pressure or cardiac conditions should consult their physicians regarding the Head Stand. (It is important to note that there are physicians in India who recommend the Head Stand as an aid in correcting these conditions. However, these judgments must be made on an individual basis.)

In regard to the completed posture (Fig. 10): eventually, we would want to be able to hold the body in an absolutely straight line, the legs aligned with the trunk as depicted. But in the beginning, simply attaining an approximate completed position is satisfactory. Come down from the position the moment you feel your balance becoming questionable. In this case, rest a few moments with your head down and make another attempt. We would like to avoid tumbling forward, so if you begin to lose your balance, keep the weight of your legs toward your chest and you will come down in the right direction.

We have recommended a maximum of three minutes in the completed posture. This time can be gradually increased—a few seconds each week—when you have become totally secure in the completed position for a period of three months. Be sure that your counting and timing are accurate. You can count the shorter periods of holding by mentally approximating seconds, but the longer holds should be timed with a watch or clock.

It is a wise precaution to surround yourself with a few pillows for added protection in the event you lose your balance.

Some students use the wall as an aid during their initial practice. The body is placed close to the wall and it supports the back and legs in Figs. 8 and 10. However, you should not resort to the wall as an aid until you have attempted the movements many times and are absolutely convinced that you are not making progress.

A multitude of Yoga students who in their entire lives had never inverted their bodies have accomplished the completed Head Stand with patient practice.

If you wish to add the Head Stand to your daily **Fitness Program,** you should include it following the Bow (17) in the **PM Routine** of the **Complete Program** and following the Knee and Thigh Stretch (9) in the **AM Routine** of the **Modified Program.**

(20) **lotus postures**

We sit in the cross-legged or Lotus positions when we practice a number of the techniques in this course. These ancient-seated postures were primarily developed for the practice of meditation; that is, for sitting quietly and engaging in various forms of introspection. To derive the greatest benefits from such an interval of quietude, however brief or lengthy, the mind must be fully focused on the meditation exercise. Therefore, it is essential to reduce the possibilities of distractions to a minimum. We have already recommended that your practice area should be chosen with a view to minimizing external disturbances. But of equal importance are the internal disturbances—the distractions produced by thoughts and emotions. Whenever the body moves, the mind is disturbed because the two are inseparable. If the body is uncomfortable, the mind is forced to acknowledge this discomfort; if the senses are engaged (something catches your eye, ear, etc.), you cannot concentrate. If thoughts continue to race through your mind, you cannot focus your attention in the required meditative manner. If your breathing is irregular, the mind is correspondingly disturbed. The ancient gurus were well aware of these problems and developed the Lotus postures to aid in the solution.

The Lotus, when perfected, enables you to sit for extended periods of time almost completely motionless. There is great stability in the posture. The legs are literally "locked" out of the way so that they do not continually move and distract the mind. The trunk and head are balanced and firmly supported. Further, simply sitting correctly in this posture has a remarkable quieting effect on the senses and produces an automatic slowing of the breathing rhythm. Thus the stage is set for meaningful meditation, or simply an interval of quietude to relax the emotions, senses, and mind.

Within a few weeks of beginning your Lotus practice, you should accomplish a satisfactory position. Indeed, depending upon the structure and flexibility of your legs, you may do a very respectable Half- or even Full-Lotus in your first attempt. But the degree of attainment is absolutely unimportant in the beginning stages; the essential thing is the patient practice that will lead to success. There are many benefits for the knees, ankles, and feet inherent in this practice.

(A) simple posture

People who are overweight, elderly, or exceptionally stiff may have to begin with this position until sufficient flexibility is developed in the thighs, knees, ankles, and feet.

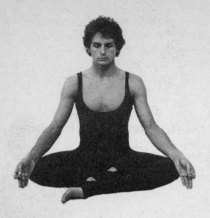

1 Cross ankles and draw heels in as far as possible.

Hold spine and head straight, but relaxed.

Rest backs of wrists on knees and touch index fingers to thumbs with slight pressure.

Lower eyelids.

Notes

You may find that your knees are raised quite some distance from the floor. They will gradually and automatically be lowered as you continue to sit in the position.

Use this position whenever a cross-legged posture is indicated in the directions for the *asanas*.

If the legs become uncomfortable, extend them straight outward; massage the knees for a few moments and then resume the position with the legs reversed, so that if the right was on top before extending the legs, the left is now on top.

Do not remain in the position longer than is comfortable (this time will increase with each sitting), and always extend the legs straight outward for a few moments before standing.

(B) half-lotus

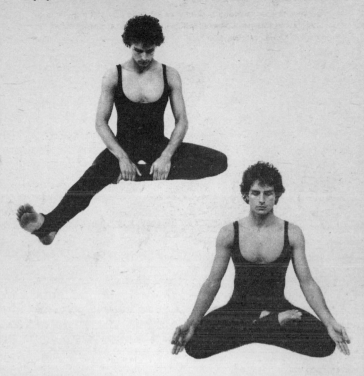

1 Extend legs.

Hands place left heel as far in as possible.

2 Hands place right foot either on left thigh or in the cleft of left leg, whichever is more comfortable.

Bring right knee as close to floor as possible.

Hold spine and head straight, but relaxed.

Rest backs of wrists on knees and touch index fingers to thumbs with slight pressure.

Lower eyelids. (Eyes are not entirely closed; a slit of light remains.)

(See Notes that follow Full-Lotus.)

(C) **full-lotus**

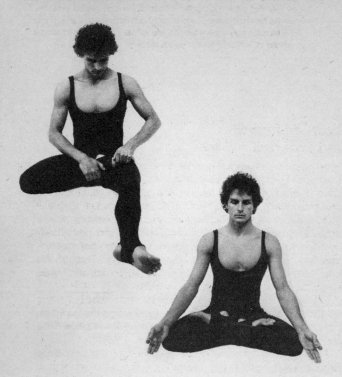

1 Extend legs.

Hands place right foot on left thigh as close to groin as possible.

If right knee will not rest on floor you cannot, at present, execute the Full-Lotus. Simply rest right forearm on right leg and sit this way for 1 to 2 minutes; then reverse legs and rest left forearm on left leg. Weight of arm will help stretch thigh so that knee may eventually rest on floor. Once knee is on floor, you can proceed to final step.

2 Hands place left foot on right thigh as close to groin as possible.

Hold spine straight, but relaxed.

Rest backs of wrists on knees and touch index fingers to thumbs with slight pressure.

Lower eyelids. (Eyes are not entirely closed; a slit of light remains.)

If discomfort is experienced, hold the position for only a few seconds. You can keep your hands on your right foot so that you may quickly remove the foot after testing the effect of the completed position. Remove the foot and extend legs straight outward. If you can get into the Full-Lotus for only a few seconds you will very shortly be holding it for a minute or more. The legs adjust quickly.

Notes for the Half- and Full-Lotus

Wherever cross-legged posture is indicated in the directions, use the Full-Lotus. If the Full-Lotus is too difficult, use the Half-Lotus. Remember that we have no wish to torture your legs. You proceed, as in all Yoga practice, cautiously, in gradual stages. If you are successful in attaining the completed positions, fine. If not, simply revert to an easier sitting position and periodically continue to attempt the more advanced. Remember that the **practice** for the Full-Lotus is of value to your legs. Through this practice they become supple, strengthened, firmed, and regain a youthful "spring."

A small pillow that provides approximately 0 inches of sitting height can be tested. This additional height raises the trunk and simultaneously lowers the knees. But do not use the pillow if it is not needed.

Although it is recommended that in the learning period the legs can be reversed in both the Half- and Full-Lotus, you should practice to eventually attain those leg positions first indicated because they are traditional for meditation and certain other techniques.

It is essential that the spine and head be erect but relaxed. The chin is aligned with the navel. The eyes are not entirely closed; a slit of light is permitted to enter at the bottom. In this manner you remain suspended between the waking and sleeping states.

Touching the tips of the index fingers to the thumbs (*mudra*) closes the circuit and retains the life-force within the body. This touching should be firm.

We caution against exhibiting the Lotus as an acrobatic accomplishment for the approval of your friends. This posture is for

121

your private practice only. Neither the Lotus nor Head Stand or, indeed, any of the *asanas* should ever be exhibited for frivolous purposes.

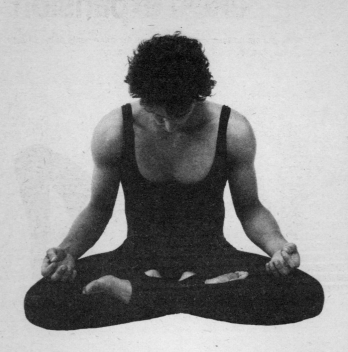

Do not:

slump or allow head to bend forward. Notice how model does not have feet drawn in as far as possible, has wrists on thighs rather than knees, has eyes completely closed instead of allowing a slit of light to enter at the bottom of the sockets, and is neglecting to exert slight pressure in touching index fingers to thumbs.

2 (A) advanced chest expansion

When you are completely comfortable in the movements of the Chest Expansion (2), cautiously attempt the following:

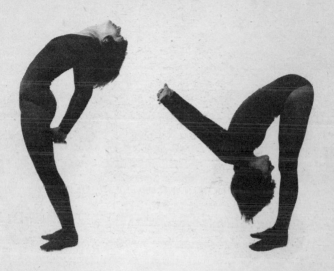

1 Slowly bend trunk backward until thumbs press against thighs.
   Eyes are open; knees straight.
   Hold for 5, as steady as possible.

2 Slowly straighten up and bend forward, bringing forehead as close to knees as possible. In extreme position, forehead touches knees.
   Bring arms over back as far as possible and keep them high.
   Hold for 10.

The Chest Expansion is a technique of the **AM Routine** in both the **Complete** and **Modified Programs.** Perform the more moderate movements, as previously practiced, once. Include the advanced movements in the second performance.

5 (A) advanced balance posture

When you are completely secure in the balance necessary for the moderate movements of the Balance Posture (5), practice to attain the following positions:

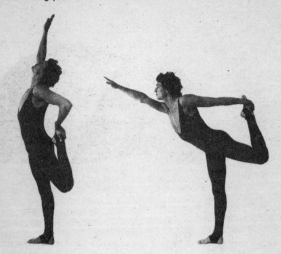

1 The foot is now brought up to the buttock or lower back.

The upraised arm moves slightly farther backward and there is a more acute curving of the spine than previously.

Hold for 5.

2 Move directly into the depicted position. Leg is brought backward as far as possible and arm comes forward. **Move very slowly.**

Hold for 5.

Slowly lower arm and leg, and perform identical movements on opposite side.

The Balance Posture is a technique of the **PM Routine** in the **Complete Program.** Perform the moderate movements as previously practiced, twice. Include the advanced movements above in the third performance. (The repetitions are alternated from right side to left side.)

7 (A) advanced back stretch

When you are able to comfortably hold your feet in the moderate movements of the Back Stretch (7), attempt to gradually attain the extreme position.

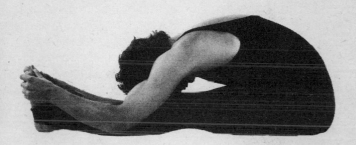

Hands hold toes.

Forehead rests on knees.

Elbows touch floor.

Knees must not bend; body is fully stretched but remains relaxed. Be constantly aware of your body's ability and never attempt to go even an inch beyond it. This ability can vary from day to day, so your practice requires total attention to each movement.

Hold for 20.

The Back Stretch is a technique of the **AM Routine** in the **Complete Program.** Perform the moderate movements as previously practiced, twice. Include the above movements in the third performance.

Notes

Lowering the elbows to the floor as depicted provides a powerful stretch for the legs and is the ultimate stretch for the back and spine. Note that it is the toes that must be held, not the feet or heels.

8 (A) advanced alternate leg stretch

When you are able to comfortably hold your foot on both sides of the Alternate Leg Stretch (8), attempt to gradually attain the extreme position.

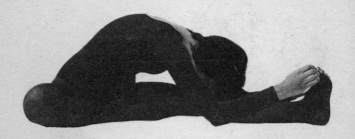

Hands hold toes.

Forehead rests on knee.

Elbows touch floor.

Knee is straight; body is fully stretched but remains relaxed.

Hold for 20.

The Alternate Leg Stretch is a technique of the **PM Routines** in both the **Complete** and **Modified Programs.** Perform the moderate movements as previously practiced, once. Include the above movements in the second performance.

Notes

Lowering the elbows to the floor as depicted provides the ultimate leg stretch and assists in firming and strengthening the lower back. When the left leg is extended, the right side of the lumbar will be emphasized and vice versa.

10 (A) advanced twist

When you have become accustomed to twisting the spine in the "corkscrew" manner of the Twist (10), substitute this technique which imparts a more intensive spinal manipulation.

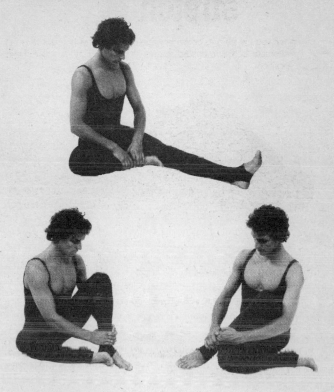

1 In a seated position, extend legs outward.
   Place right foot as depicted, with heel as far in as possible.

2 Bring left leg toward you so that you can take a firm hold of left ankle with both hands.

3 Study the photograph. You now swing left foot **over** right knee and place sole firmly on floor adjacent to right thigh.

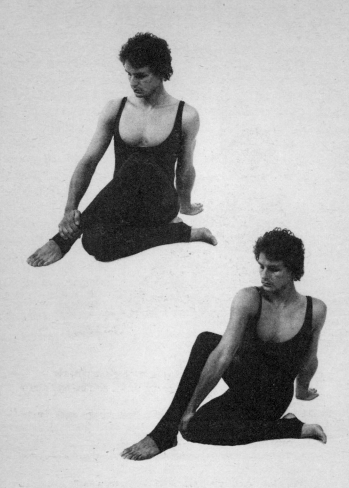

4 Remove left hand from ankle and place it firmly on floor behind back for support.

5 Remove right hand from ankle and slowly bring it **over** left leg.

Take a firm hold on right knee with right hand. (Some adjustment of the leg and trunk may be necessary to accomplish this position.)

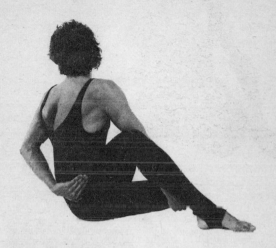

6 Very slowly turn trunk and head as far to the **left** as possible.

Simultaneously, move left hand from the floor to hold the right side of waist.

Head is turned as far to left as possible. Trunk remains erect. Breathe normally.

Hold without motion for 10.

Place left palm on floor and slowly turn trunk forward so that you are in position of Fig. 5.

Relax a few moments and repeat the twisting movement.

Perform 3 times.

Return trunk to forward position and extend legs.

Perform identical movements on opposite side by carefully exchanging words *right* and *left* in above directions.

Perform 3 times to left, then 3 times to right.

The Twist is a technique of the **AM Routines** in both the **Complete** and **Modified Programs.** When you have mastered the Advanced Twist, substitute it for the previous movements.

Notes

At first, the positions of Figs. 5 and 6 may feel cramped. The body will soon adjust to them.

Be sure that the twist is as complete as possible by turning the head far to the side as though the chin would touch the shoulder. The hand has a firm hold on the waist which aids the spine in twisting.

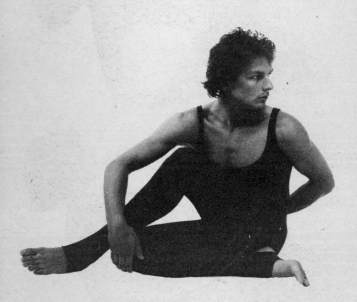

Do not:

slump or neglect to turn head as far as possible to side. Notice how model has reached **around** the knee rather than **over** it, does not have sole of foot fully on floor, and is simply resting hand on back rather than firmly holding opposite side of waist.

11 (A) advanced backward bend

When you are completely comfortable in Fig. 5 of the Backward Bend (11), attempt to gradually attain these advanced positions.

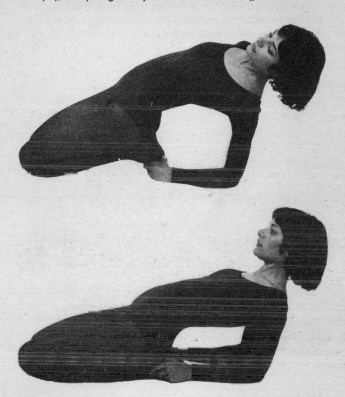

1 Very slowly and cautiously lower either elbow to floor.

2 Very slowly and cautiously lower other elbow to floor.
Hold feet.

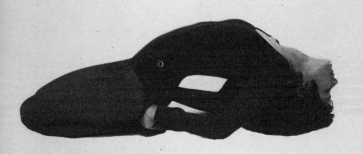

3 Very slowly and cautiously lower top of head to floor.

Relax as much as possible to make the hold easier.

Hold for 10.

Very slowly and cautiously raise head several inches. Place either palm firmly on floor. Push up so that other palm may also be placed on floor. Slowly raise trunk and proceed to come into a seated position.

The Backward Bend is a technique of the **AM Routine** in the **Complete Program.** Perform the first position of the Backward Bend (feet rest on floor) as previously practiced, once. The second position previously practiced (toes rest on floor), together with these advanced movements, constitute the second performance.

Notes

All movements must be attempted very slowly and cautiously. Lowering one elbow to the floor may be all that you can accomplish for several practice sessions. In this case, simply hold that position for the count of 10 and come out of the position. Gradually, the body will adjust and you can then proceed to lowering the other elbow. As always, there is no hurry to attain the extreme position, and absolutely no strain should be experienced.

13 (A) advanced plough

When you are completely comfortable in the first position of the Plough (13), practice to attain the following 2 additional positions:

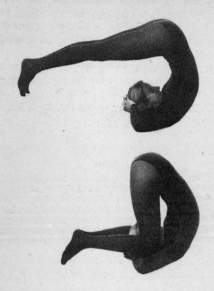

1 Upon completing the holding count of 20 for the first position, bring hands up and clasp them on top of head.

Inch feet backward as far as possible.

Knees straight, chin pressed tightly against chest.

Hold for 20.

2 Slowly and cautiously lower knees to touch the floor within the arms.

Hold for 20.

Come out of the position exactly as previously practiced.

When these 2 advanced positions have been accomplished, perform the sequence of the 3 positions twice.

Notes

The position of the Plough that was previously performed places the emphasis in the lumbar area, the lower spine. The position of Fig. 1 in these advanced movements transfers the emphasis to the middle area of the back and spine, and the position of Fig. 2 emphasizes the upper area and the cervical vertebrae. In this way, the back and spine receive a thorough workout with the movements of the Plough.

At first, because of the way in which the chin is pressed against the chest, breathing may be impeded. Again, the body and lungs adjust to these positions within several practice sessions and breathing will not be a problem, particularly if you consciously slow its rhythm.

Surprisingly, the position of Fig. 2, which appears to be contorted and difficult, is actually one of the most relaxing of the *asanas*! Once attained, it provides a wonderful tension-relieving stretch without further effort. In this position the body feels almost weightless.

part 2

techniques included in the *special routines*

The additional techniques (21–29) that follow are those that because of time limitations, are not included in the **Fitness Programs,** but become extremely useful when dealing with particular situations and problems.

In undertaking the **Special Routines** of this section, you will be performing selections of the techniques learned in Part 1 and, in certain cases, including one or more of these additional *asanas* and *pranayama*. Therefore, you need not at this point learn and practice all of these nine Special Techniques, but utilize only those which are indicated in the **Special Routines** that you elect to perform. However, if in experimenting with any of these techniques you find them particularly helpful, you can certainly include them in your regular **Fitness Program.**

(21) roll twist

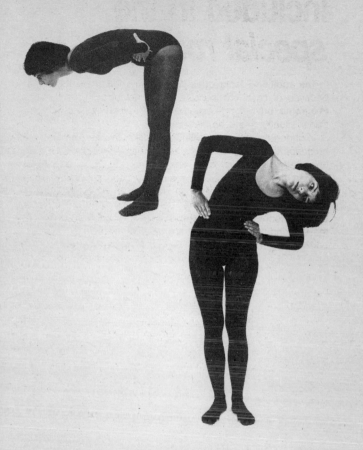

1 Stand erect with legs together and hands on hips.
  Bend trunk forward to position depicted.

2 Slowly roll and twist trunk to left side. (Trunk does not simply bend to
  side; it rolls and twists in slow motion.)
  Hold for 2.

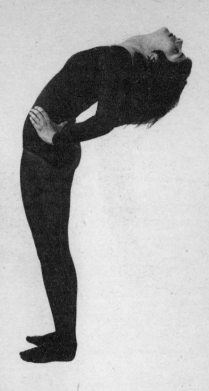

3 Slowly roll and twist trunk to backward position.

Hold for 2.

Slowly roll and twist trunk to right side.

Hold for 2.

Slowly roll and twist trunk to frontward position of Fig. 1.

This completes 1 round. Repeat.

Following final repetition, slowly straighten to upright position and lower arms to sides.

Perform 5 rounds counterclockwise and 5 rounds clockwise.

(22) leg clasp

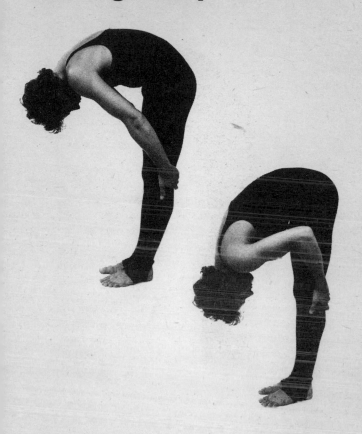

1 In a standing position with feet together, very slowly bend forward and
   firmly hold backs of knees.

2 Very slowly and cautiously lower trunk as far as possible without strain.
   Knees straight, neck relaxed, head down.
   Hold without motion for 10.
   Relax and return trunk to position of Fig. 1.

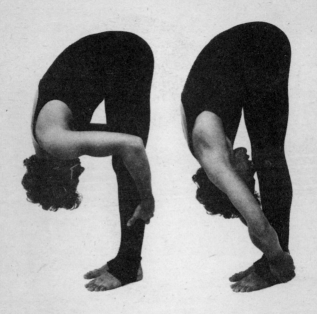

3 Move hands down from knees and firmly hold calves.

Bracing hands against calves, slowly and cautiously lower trunk as far as possible.

Hold for 10.

Relax and very slowly straighten to the upright position.

4 This is the advanced position that results from practice. Hands now hold ankles and head touches legs. Hold for 10. If attained, this position is to be substituted for the calves position.

Perform once in the knees position and once in the calves or ankles position. (Remember that regardless of how flexible or strong you feel on any given day, the first performance of an *asana* is always in an elementary, moderate position because you cannot know the actual condition of your body on that day.)

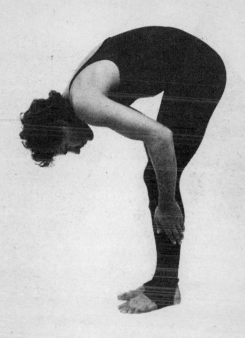

Do not:

place hands against (rather than firmly hold) legs, bend knees, or keep neck rigid.

(23) leg over

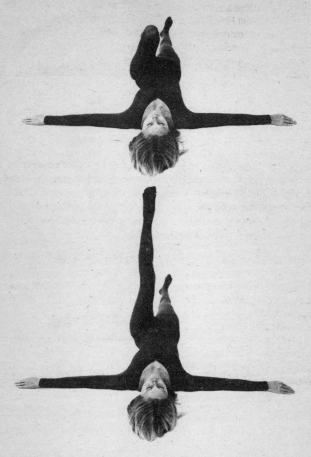

1 Lying on your back, stretch arms outward at chest level. Palms rest on floor.

Bend left knee and bring it toward abdomen.

2 Slowly extend leg straight upward.

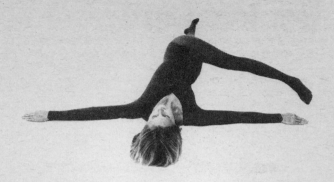

3 Slowly bring leg over to right side.

Slowly lower leg as far as possible. Touch foot to floor if possible.

Entire back must remain on floor; do not roll trunk. Keep left leg parallel with arm; do not lower it.

Hold without motion for 5.

Return left leg to position of Fig. 2 and slowly lower it to floor.

Execute identical movements with right leg.

Perform 5 times with each leg, alternating from left to right.

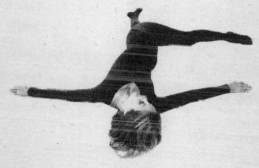

Do not:

permit back to leave floor, lower arms from chest level, lower leg so that it is not parallel with outstretched arm. (If foot cannot touch floor, simply hold it at its lowest position for the count of 5.)

(24) side raise

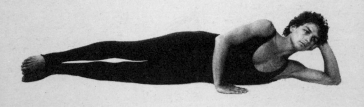

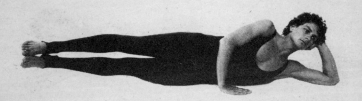

1 Lie on left side with left elbow positioned as illustrated. Rest side of head and ear in palm. Right hand is placed firmly on floor adjacent to abdomen.

2 Push against floor with hand and slowly raise legs several inches from floor. (Legs remain together and must not sway to front or back.)

Hold as steady as possible for 10.

Slowly lower legs to floor.

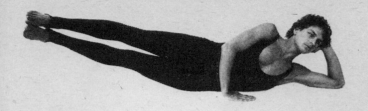

3 Now raise legs as high as possible.

Hold without motion for 10.

Slowly lower legs to floor.

Repeat.

Execute identical movements lying on right side.

Perform 3 times on each side—once in the moderate position and twice in the extreme position.

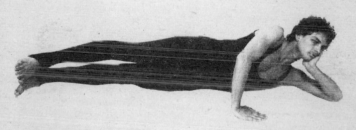

Do not:

place supporting hand on chin, cheek, allow legs to sway to front or back, place hand away from abdomen.

(25) **back push-up**

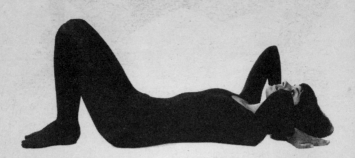

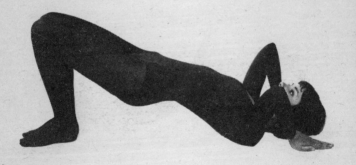

1 Lying on your back, rest palms on floor adjacent to head, fingers pointing toward rear. Heels are drawn in toward buttocks, soles rest on floor; knees and feet are together.

2 Brace feet and fingers against floor and raise body a moderate distance.

Hold as steady as possible for 10.

Slowly lower body to floor.

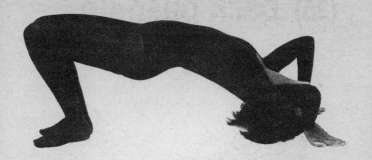

3 Now raise as high as possible.

Hold for 10.

Slowly lower body to floor.

Repeat.

Perform 3 times—once in the moderate position and twice in the extreme position.

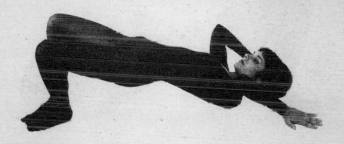

Do not:

move hands away from head, ooparate fingers or knees.

(26) charging breath

This breathing technique introduces an increased supply of *prana* into the lungs in a rapid manner and literally "charges" the organism.

If you have performed the Abdominal Lift, you will have gained control over the distension and contraction movements that are necessary. If you have not practiced these movements, you must do so now. Turn to the Abdominal Lift (18) and learn the movements described for Figs. 1 and 2.

These distending-contracting movements are now combined with breathing in the following manner:

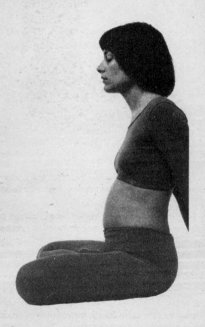

1 Seated in a cross-legged posture, inhale and simultaneously **distend** the abdomen. (Be sure you distend; that is, push the abdomen out when inhaling. Your initial tendency may be to contract the abdomen when inhaling but this is incorrect.)

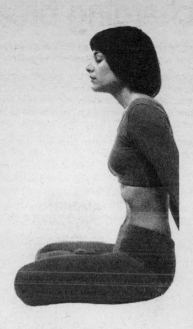

2 Without pause, quickly and forcefully **contract** the abdomen so that the air is forced from the lungs and you execute an inhalation through the nose.

Without pause, distend the abdomen and inhale; without pause, contract the abdomen and exhale, and continue this process.

Perform 25 times during the learning period and 50 times when you have perfected the technique. Following the final repetition, perform 1 Complete Breath as previously learned (1B).

Perform the 25–50 movements 5 times so that you do a total of from 125 to 250 breaths. (An inhalation and exhalation constitute one breath.) Perform 1 Complete Breath following each group of 25–50. Begin the next round immediately following the Complete Breath; do not pause or rest. Upon completion of the final Complete Breath, relax but remain quietly seated in the cross-legged posture for approximately 1 minute. Your eyelids may be lowered throughout the movements.

151

Notes

As pointed out above, there may be an initial tendency to coordinate the breathing and abdominal movements in the exact opposite manner than that indicated in the directions. If this is the case, you must simply practice the movements slowly and attentively until they are mastered. Once the coordination has been perfected, practice to make the movements and the breathing rhythmic and crisp. In the beginning stages you can distend and contract the abdomen slowly and in an exaggerated fashion. But as control is gained, the movements of the abdomen are minimized and each breath is greatly accelerated so that the combined inhalation and exhalation can be executed in half a second. When full control is achieved, the 250 movements, together with the Complete Breaths, can be performed in 2–3 minutes. At that point you may find it easy to do 100 rather than 50 breaths to each round, making a total of 500 rather than 250. But you must build to this slowly and never sacrifice the precise and rhythmic movements for speed.

This technique not only charges the organism but has a cleansing effect on the respiratory system. It requires effort to learn and perform the Charging Breath correctly, but this effort will be well rewarded. Do the best you can at each practice session and you will soon catch on to the knack of the necessary coordination. Giving up on the technique because it is not mastered during the first few practice sessions is a grave error.

As you sit quietly, following completion of the final round, you will experience clarity of mind and an elevated state of consciousness.

(27) alternate nostril breathing

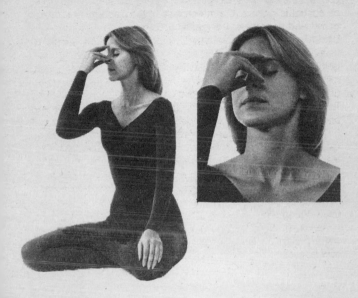

1 Sit in a cross-legged posture and rest left hand on left knee.

Study the photograph. Place tip of right thumb lightly against right nostril and the ring and little fingers lightly against the left. The index and middle fingers are together and rest with light pressure between the eyebrows. When the technique has been learned, lower the eyelids.

Exhale fully through both nostrils.

2 Close **right** nostril by pressing thumb firmly against it.

Inhale through the **left** nostril and fill the lungs during a slow, rhythmic count of 8.

153

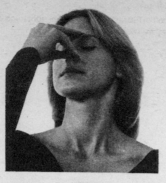

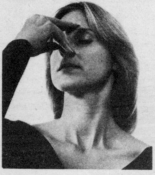

3 Close the **left** nostril with the ring finger so that **both** nostrils are now closed.

Retain the air for a rhythmic count of 4.

4 Release the **right** nostril (the **left** remains closed) and exhale fully through the **right** nostril during a slow, rhythmic count of 8.

Without pause:

Inhale through the **right** nostril (the same nostril through which you just exhaled) during a slow, rhythmic count of 8.

Close the **right** nostril (**both** nostrils are now closed) and retain the air for a count of 4.

Open the **left** nostril (the **right** remains closed) and exhale fully through the **left** nostril during a slow, rhythmic count of 8.

This completes one round. **Without pause,** repeat by inhaling through the **left** nostril, and continue.

Upon completion of the final round, rest the right hand on the right knee and sit quietly for at least 1 minute.

Perform 7 rounds.

Notes

Alternate Nostril Breathing acts as a profound natural tranquilizer. There are very few emotional or mental disturbances that do not respond to this technique. Its effectiveness is due to the way in which it regulates the *prana* that enters the organism through the nose: the positive-negative ratio is equalized. In advanced Yoga, Alternate Nostril Breathing is utilized—in a more elaborate application—as a principal technique in cleansing the subtle nervous system (*nadis*) and arousing the primal latent power (*kundalini*).

All breathing must be performed quietly and deeply. The air is to be felt more in the throat than in the nose and it must at no point "gush" or "hiss" in or out. The raised hand is relaxed, and the spine and head are held erect but also relaxed. The eyelids should be lowered (not closed).

The uninterrupted, rhythmic count, 8—4—8, is crucial and must be carefully attended to. Set a steady beat in your mind and concentrate totally on the counting; **do not permit the breathing to become automatic while your mind wanders.**

This technique has also proven most helpful to those suffering with nasal congestion. In these cases, it is usually not possible to breathe "quietly," but this should not deter practice. A clearing of the passages is usually noted several minutes following completion of the exercise.

That period during which you sit quietly (following the final round) can be one of the most elevating of the day.

Summary:

Exhale deeply	
Inhale through left	count 8
Retain (both closed)	count 4
Exhale through right	count 8
Inhale through right	count 8
Retain (both closed)	count 4
Exhale through left	count 8

This completes 1 round.

(28) **deep relaxation**

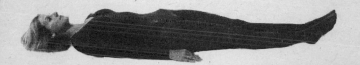

Lie on your back, arms at sides in the most comfortable position. Allow body to become limp.

Focus attention on your feet: if they are tensed in any way, relax them.

Next, become aware of your calves and knees; relax them completely.

Determine if all the muscles in your thighs are relaxed.

Slowly draw your consciousness up into the lower abdomen, then the upper abdomen, then the chest. As you become aware of each of these areas, make sure there are no muscular contractions.

Now shift your attention to your fingers, then the lower arms, upper arms, and shoulders. Feel the condition of each in turn and withdraw all support so that they are absolutely limp.

Next, determine if your neck is in the most comfortable position; if not, adjust it.

Finally, relax your jaw and face. Close eyes.

Become aware that your entire body is now in a state of deep relaxation. Exclude all thoughts and concentrate on your breathing. Continue to observe your breathing for as long as you wish.

(29) direction of the life-force

In Hatha Yoga, health and well-being are defined in terms of an adequate supply and the normal circulation of *prana*, life-force. It is partially to help ensure these that Hatha Yoga is practiced. If the *pranic* supply is reduced, or its circulation impeded, various negative conditions develop, and health is impaired accordingly. All healing, regardless of the method, or by whom it is applied, is a conscious or unconscious effort to normalize the *pranic* flow.

In this technique, *prana* is consciously directed to any area where a negative condition exists. The premise is that by increasing the supply of life-force at the point where it is needed, healing is promoted.

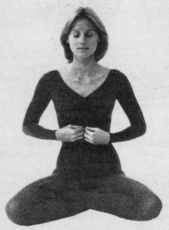

1 Sit in a cross-legged posture. Once the directions are understood, it will be necessary to have the eyes entirely closed for purposes of visualization.

Let us assume that you are experiencing tension, stiffness, and general discomfort in your left shoulder. It is into this area, therefore, that you wish to direct increased *prana*.

Place all 10 fingertips lightly on the solar plexus. This is the area located at the top of the abdomen, beneath the ribs, where *prana* collects during respiration. Exhale fully.

Very slowly inhale deeply and fully. During the inhalation, visualize the *pranic* current as an intense white light. It enters through your nostrils, moves downward into the region of your solar plexus, and passes into your fingertips where it remains. This must be the continuous visualization during the entire *slow* inhalation.

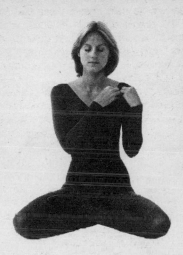

2 When the inhalation is completed, **retain the air** and transfer your 10 fingertips to that area of your shoulder where the discomfort is experienced.

Very slowly exhale deeply and fully. During this exhalation, visualize the *prana*, the white light, flowing from your fingertips into your shoulder, flooding it with life-force. This is the continuous visualization during the entire **slow** exhalation.

When the exhalation is completed, suspend breathing for a few moments while you slowly return your fingertips to the solar plexus.

Begin the next inhalation and repeat the procedure.

Upon completion of the final repetition, rest your hands on your knees, breathe normally, and become acutely aware of what is transpiring within.

Perform 7 times.

Notes

Obviously, your attention must be fully focused on the visualization of the white light throughout the exercise. If the light is slow in manifesting, persevere in your attempts; it will come. If the white light fades, or is entirely lost, remanifest it by an intensified visualization effort. If your attention wanders, return it gently but firmly to the imagery.

If, after the first group of seven, you wish to perform additional repetitions to increase the possibility of remedying the shoulder (or any other) condition, you should certainly do so. You can rest briefly following the first group of seven and then perform two additional groups, making a total of twenty-one. Additionally, you can repeat the practice at various times of the day or night.

Although we have used the shoulder as an example, *prana* may be directed to any part of the body. If an area of your back is afflicted, perform the inhalation as indicated above and then separate your hands and bring them around to the pertinent area during retention of the air. During the exhalation, the white light is directed into that area; return your fingertips to the solar plexus during suspension of breathing, and repeat the process. In the case of a headache, the fingertips are transferred to the forehead, etc.

If, during an illness, you are unable to assume the cross-legged posture, the technique can be practiced in a reclining position. With a little consideration, you will be able to make whatever adjustments are necessary in almost any situation to accommodate the technique.

Practice to make the flow of the white light steady and strong. As you continue to gain aptitude in visualization, the effectiveness of the technique will increase.

special-situation routines

In addition to their utilization as an effective form of physical therapy (which is the subject of the **Special Problems** section that follows), the Yoga techniques can serve as ever-present aids in many everyday circumstances. Of the special situations about which the author's readers and television viewers have requested information, there are two that currently command the greatest interest: (1) sports, (2) preparing for an important event such as an examination, interview, performance, meeting, etc. Accordingly, this section presents routines that can be advantageously applied in these two situations. The routines are the result of reports from numerous athletes, students, and business and professional people who have undertaken to experiment with the Yoga programs we have suggested.

If you have attained the advanced positions, include them in the routines as indicated. If you are not yet ready for the advanced positions, simply disregard the references.

As you become increasingly familiar with the effects of the various *asanas* in your **Fitness Program,** you will, if necessary, be able to design a program to meet your personal, special-situation needs. But remember that all such routines are **supplemental** and must not be considered as substitutes for the **Fitness Program.**

sports

This section consists of two routines. The first is for practice immediately **before** participation in a sporting event and is designed to increase enjoyment and proficiency. The *asanas*, together with the Charging Breath, provide a quick loosening of the spine, joints, and limbs, and will assist in increasing endurance and concentration.

The second routine is for practice as soon as possible **after** the event. The indicated *asanas*, together with Deep Relaxation, will help prevent or relieve tension, soreness, tightness, fatigue, and other negative effects that can occur from the various types of stress inherent in sports.

Each routine can be performed in approximately seven minutes.

Before

chest expansion
(2) basic techniques; (2A) advanced techniques

Perform twice: once in the moderate position and once in your extreme position. Hold the backward bends for 5 and the forward bends for 10.

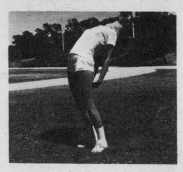

twist
(10) basic techniques; (10A) advanced techniques

Perform 3 times on each side: once in the moderate position and twice in your extreme position. Hold each twist for 5.

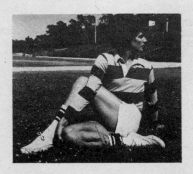

alternate leg stretch
(8) basic techniques; (8A) advanced techniques

Perform twice with each leg: once in the moderate position and once in your extreme position. Hold each stretch for 20.

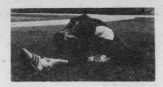

bow
(17) basic techniques; (17A) advanced techniques

Perform 3 times: once in the moderate position and twice in your extreme position. Hold each raise for 10.

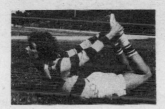

charging breath
(26) special techniques

Perform 5 rounds of 25–50 breaths per round. Follow each round with 1 Complete Breath.

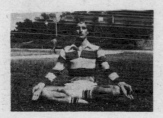

After

shoulder stand
(12) basic techniques

Perform once. Hold 1–3 minutes.

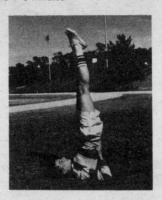

cobra
(14) basic techniques

Perform twice: once in the moderate position and once in your extreme position. Hold each raise for 20.

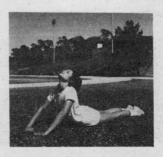

neck movements
(15) basic techniques

Perform the 3 movements twice. Hold each for 10.

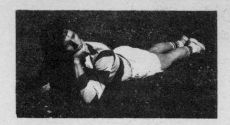

back stretch
(7) basic techniques; (7A) advanced techniques

Perform twice: once in the moderate position and once in your extreme position. Hold each stretch for 20.

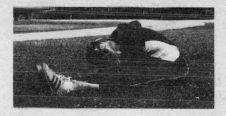

deep relaxation
(28) special techniques

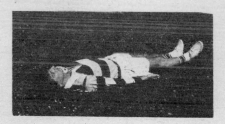

Prior to an important meeting, examination, interview, or any encounter that requires particular alertness and the absence of tension or anxiety.

This routine consists of three previously learned *asanas* and Alternate Nostril Breathing, a breathing technique that has a profoundly quieting effect on the emotions, enabling one's attention to be fully concentrated on the matter at hand.

The routine requires approximately seven minutes of privacy; it can be performed prior to leaving home or in any private situation that may be available immediately prior to the encounter. If the routine cannot be undertaken, a series of Complete Breaths (1B, Basic Techniques) performed in a regular seated position, without the raising of the shoulders, will prove helpful.

chest expansion
(2) basic techniques; (2A) advanced techniques

Perform twice: once in the moderate position and once in your extreme position. Hold the backward bends for 5 and the forward bends for 10.

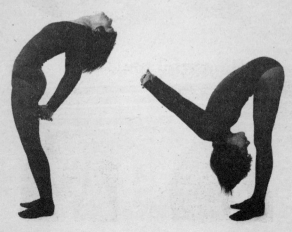

back stretch
(7) basic techniques; (7A) advanced techniques

Perform twice: once in the moderate position and once in your extreme position. Hold each stretch for 20.

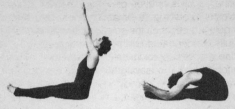

cobra
(14) basic techniques

Perform twice: once in the moderate position and once in your extreme position. Hold each raise for 10.

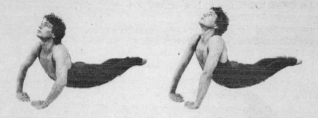

alternate nostril breathing
(27) special techniques

Perform 7 rounds

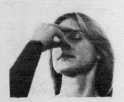
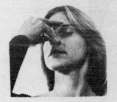

special-problem routines

Many physical and emotional problems have responded in a highly favorable manner to Yoga practice. The following pages contain those routines which, in the author's extensive experience with Yoga as a therapeutic agent, have proven effective for the indicated problems. These routines are not suggested as an alternative to professional treatment; rather, with the approval of the therapist, they offer an approach that can work to great advantage in conjunction with the general treatment that has been prescribed.

There are three ways of utilizing these routines:

1. Include them in the **Fitness Program.** In this case, you may have to increase or decrease the number of repetitions and the holding time indicated in Part 1 because of the different instructions for the **Problem Routines.** You will also have to incorporate into the **Fitness Program** the **Special Techniques** that are indicated. Therefore, if you elect to incorporate one or more of the **Problem Routines** into your **Fitness Program,** it will be necessary to lengthen both the AM and PM sessions, and you must be prepared to spend additional time in practice. It will also be necessary for you to carefully design your own program in accordance with the above considerations.

2. Perform the **Problem Routine** you select in a practice session that is separate from the AM and PM **Fitness Program** sessions. If more than one **Problem Routine** is undertaken, you can perform them on alternate days, or rotate them over a period of several days.

3. Substitute the **Problem Routines** for the **Fitness Program.** This is the least desirable of the three possibilities and is suggested only in the event that your time for practice is extremely limited.

The photographs in the **Problem Routines** serve to remind you of the necessary movements. However, be sure to refer to the appropriate directions, photographs, and Notes of the *asanas* until you are entirely certain of what is involved. Remember that you must carefully note the number of repetitions and the holding time for the techniques of the **Problem Routines** because they are not necessarily the same as those given in Part 1 and in the instructions for the **Special Techniques.** If you have attained any of the advanced positions, include them in the routines as indicated. If you are not yet ready for the advanced positions, simply disregard the references.

In a holistic approach to fitness—which includes dealing with physical, emotional, and mental problems—nutrition plays an indispensable role. Therefore, we urge that with the approval of your physician, you adopt the Yoga nutrition principles in conjunction with the Hatha Yoga program. The pertinent information will be found in *Weight Control Through Yoga**

Weight Control Through Yoga, Richard Hittleman, Bantam Books, 1971.

abdomen
(strengthened, firmed, reduced, raised)

abdominal lift
(18) basic techniques. Standing position only

Once this technique has been mastered, practice to perform at least 10 lifts to each exhalation, so that you are performing at least 50–100 movements in each session. The number of lifts to each exhalation can exceed 10 as proficiency increases.

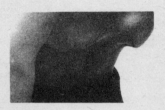

roll twist
(21) special techniques

Perform 5 rounds counterclockwise and 5 rounds clockwise.

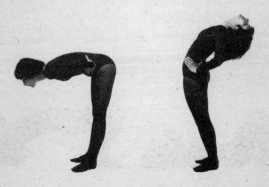

locust
(16) basic techniques

Perform 3 times: once in the moderate position and twice in your extreme position. Hold each raise for a count of 5–10.

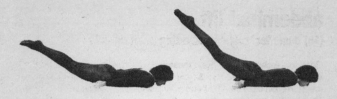

side raise
(24) special techniques

Perform 5 times each side: once in the moderate position and 4 times in your extreme position. Hold each raise for 10.

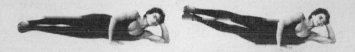

back push-up
(25) special techniques

Perform 5 times: once in the moderate position and 4 times in your extreme position. Hold each raise for 10.

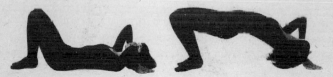

leg over
(23) special techniques

Perform your extreme position 3 times to each side, alternating from left leg to right leg. Hold each for 10.

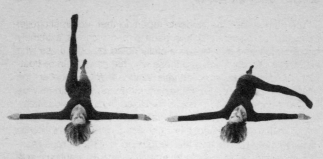

shoulder stand
(12) basic techniques

Perform once. Initially hold 1–3 minutes. As the position becomes increasingly comfortable hold 3–10 minutes.

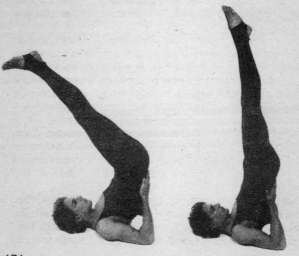

arthritis
(joint conditions and exceptional stiffness)

The number of Yoga students reporting that a dramatic relief from arthritic discomforts has been experienced is extremely encouraging and should be carefully noted by both those who suffer with this condition and those who are involved in its treatment. As you may know, arthritis victims seldom recover; the condition slowly worsens. If they are fortunate, the pain may be kept to a minimum and possibly localized through various treatments. More often, however, the pain becomes more acute and the condition does spread. Our extensive observations of arthritis victims who have applied the suggested routine of Yoga techniques leads us to conclude that this type of cautious self-manipulation can be highly effective and, in conjunction with adaptation of the Yoga nutrition principles, may constitute a cure.

One who is suffering with arthritis, bursitis, exceptional stiffness, and similar ailments is usually reluctant to "exercise" because of the pain inherent in the movements. But with Yoga we have an entirely different situation. The thorough and cautious manipulations, together with the precise **holds,** enable the practitioner to have complete control of each movement, and the slow motion minimizes or eliminates discomfort.

In the following routine, which emphasizes the joints, you can begin by moving only a few inches; any position is satisfactory. Although holding time and number of repetitions are indicated, you should discontinue the **hold** or terminate the repetitions the moment discomfort is experienced. At the next practice session, do the best you can again. In this way you will progress slowly but surely. There may be days on which your movements will be extremely limited, but this is natural and to be expected. If you understand that the difficult days are part of the improvement process and that progress consists of taking a few steps forward and one backward, you will not become impatient or discouraged.

Diet plays a crucial role, and application of the Yoga nutrition principles, including brief intervals of fasting, must be seriously considered. Such things as the elimination of dairy foods (with the possible exception of small amounts of nonfat milk and low-fat yogurt), processed foods, artificial sweeteners, and refined-sugar products together with a significant increase in raw vegetables and their juices, and fresh fruits and their juices are recommended. This information is contained in the book previously noted. (All recommendations are subject to the approval of your physician.)

The photographs in this routine depict very moderate positions of the recommended *asanas* and will serve as examples of how the other techniques of the **Fitness Program** can be performed by those who have arthritis, bursitis, etc. All movements are to be executed very cautiously, and all positions and holding times are to be modified as necessary.

chest expansion
(2) basic techniques

Perform twice. Hold the backward bends for 5 and the forward bends for 5–10.

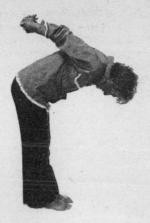

knee and thigh stretch
(9) basic techniques

Perform 3 times. Hold each stretch for 10.

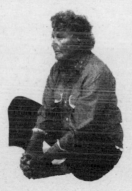

twist
(10) basic techniques

Perform twice on each side. Hold each twist for 10.

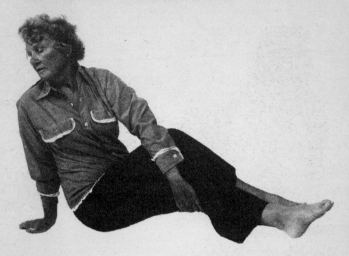

back stretch
(7) basic techniques

Perform twice. Hold each stretch for 10.

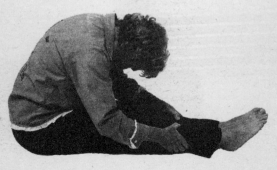

cobra
(14) basic techniques

Perform twice. Hold each raise for 10.

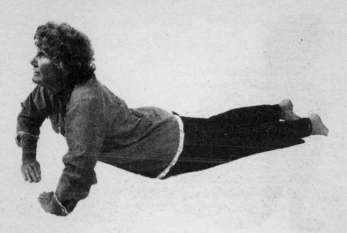

neck movements
(15) basic techniques

Perform the 3 positions twice. Hold each position for 10.

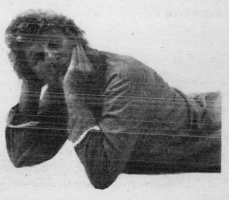

back and spine
(all areas strengthened, firmed—stiffness and tension relieved)

Although the back and spine are involved in all *asanas* of the **Fitness Programs,** the techniques of this routine are especially valuable for the objectives listed above. Problems of the back and spine are so numerous and complex that we can make no predictions as to how a specific condition will respond to the postures. However, it has been our extensive experience that this routine will accomplish those things listed above, and that it could have a favorable effect in your particular problem. More than any form of self-therapy of which we are aware, Yoga has improved or cured conditions of the back and spine.

Obtain the approval of your physician for the practice of the routine and proceed intelligently and cautiously, making progress in gradual stages.

chest expansion
(2) basic techniques; (2A) advanced techniques

Perform twice: once in the moderate position and once in your extreme position. Hold the backward bends for 10 and the forward bends for 20.

rishi's posture
(3) basic techniques

Perform the moderate position once on each side and your extreme position once on each side. Hold each position for 10.

 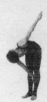

leg clasp
(22) special techniques

Perform twice: once in the moderate position and once in your extreme position. Hold each stretch for 10.

twist
(10) basic techniques; (10A) advanced techniques

Perform 3 times: once in the moderate position and twice in your extreme position. Hold each twist for 10.

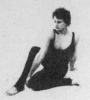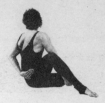

backward bend
(11) basic techniques; (11A) advanced techniques

Perform twice: once in the moderate position and once in your extreme position. Hold each bend for 20.

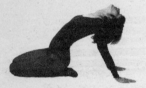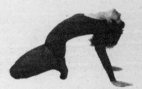

cobra
(14) basic techniques

Perform twice: once in the moderate position and once in your extreme position. Hold each raise for 20.

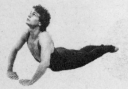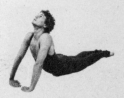

bow
(17) basic techniques

Perform 3 times: once in the moderate position and twice in your extreme position. Hold each raise for 10.

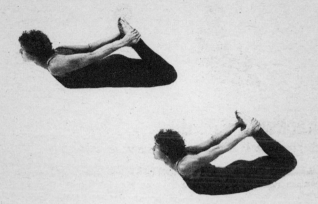

plough
(13) basic techniques; (13A) advanced techniques

Perform each of the 3 positions once. If unable to attain the 3 positions, perform your extreme position twice. Hold each position for 20.

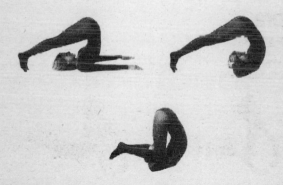

constipation

The **Fitness Program,** in conjunction with application of the Yoga nutrition principles, should greatly assist in this problem. The Abdominal Lift is an excellent technique to emphasize and can be practiced several times during the day. You must not have eaten for at least ninety minutes prior to this practice, but it can be helpful to drink half a glass of cool water five minutes before beginning the movements.

abdominal lift
(18) advanced techniques

Perform in sitting–standing sequence.

Seated: 10 lifts to each of the 5 exhalations so that you perform 50 lifts.

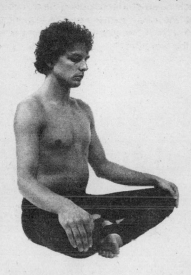

Standing: at least 10 lifts to each exhalation so that you are performing a minimum of 50 additional lifts. As proficiency increases in the standing position you can perform 25 or more lifts to each of the 5 exhalations.

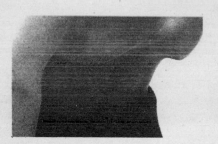

headaches

alternate nostril breathing
(27) special techniques

Perform 7 rounds.

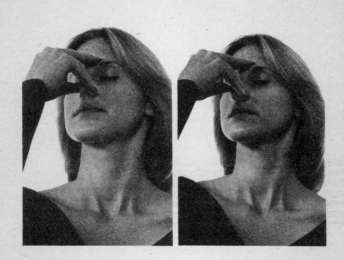

deep relaxation
(28) special techniques

Perform as indicated in the instructions.

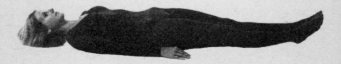

direction of the life-force
(29) special techniques

When the state of deep relaxation has been attained from the previous technique, perform the Life-Force movements, directing the *prana* into the forehead. That is, the fingertips are transferred from the solar plexus to the forehead, and during the exhalation the white light is visualized as infusing that area.

Perform 7 times.

insomnia

This is a condition which, in Yoga, we alleviate by relieving physical tension, quieting the mind and emotions, and consciously achieving the state of deep relaxation. The following routine is to be performed immediately prior to retiring.

cobra
(14) basic techniques

Perform twice: once in the moderate position and once in your extreme position. Hold each raise for 20.

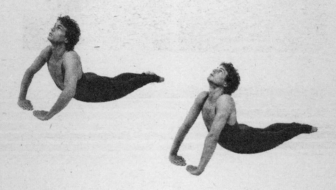

neck movements
(15) basic techniques

Perform the 3 movements twice. Hold each position for 10.

alternate nostril breathing
(27) special techniques

Perform 7 rounds.

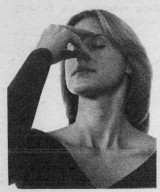 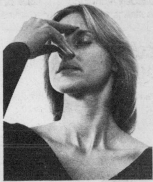

deep relaxation
(28) special techniques

Perform as indicated in the instructions. Both Alternate Nostril Breathing and Deep Relaxation can be performed in bed.

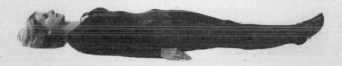

Restful sleep is a critical element of well-being. The above routine should provide the assistance one needs in the insomnia problem. (Do not eat or drink for at least two hours prior to retiring. Food must be digested. If the digestive process is occurring, the body cannot be in that state which is conducive to restful sleep.)

legs
(calves, knees, and thighs—firmed, strengthened, and revitalized—tension and stiffness relieved)

Because there are fifteen techniques that can be effectively applied, they are grouped into two routines. Both routines can be performed in one session (if time permits), or each can be practiced on alternate days: Routine 1—Monday, Routine 2—Tuesday, Routine 1—Wednesday, and so forth. In the latter case, keep a written record of which routine you should be doing during a particular practice session.

Routine 1

triangle
(4) basic techniques

Perform 3 times, alternating sides: once in the moderate position on each side and twice in your extreme position on each side. Hold each bend for 10.

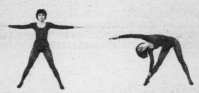

knee and thigh stretch
(9) basic techniques

Perform 3 times. Hold each stretch for 10.

locust
(16) basic techniques

Perform 3 times: once in the moderate position and twice in your extreme
position. Hold each raise for 10.

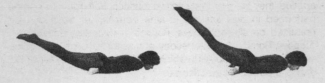

bow
(17) basic techniques

Perform 3 times: once in the moderate position and twice in your extreme
position. Hold each raise for 10.

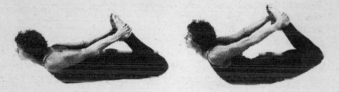

backward bend
(11) basic techniques; (11A) advanced techniques

Perform once in the moderate position with tops of feet on floor and once
in your extreme position with toes on floor. Hold each for 20.

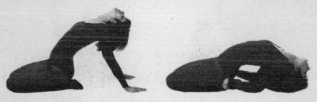

plough
(13) basic techniques; (13A) advanced techniques

If possible, perform once in each of the 3 positions; otherwise, perform twice in whatever positions you can attain. "Twice" means that you perform your position(s) once and then repeat that sequence. Hold each for 20.

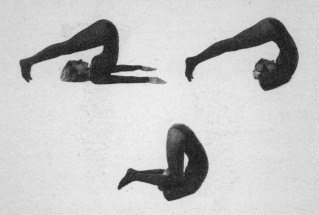

lotus
(20) advanced techniques

Use the cross-legged postures as indicated.

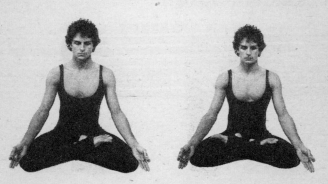

dancer's movements
(6) basic techniques

Perform 5 times. Hold on toes for 5.

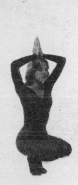
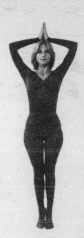

leg clasp
(22) special techniques

Perform twice: once in the moderate position and once in your extreme position. Hold each stretch for 10.

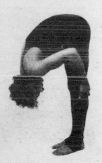
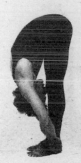

alternate leg stretch
(8) basic techniques; (8A) advanced techniques

Perform 3 times with each leg: once in the moderate position and twice in your extreme position with left leg, then same with right leg. Hold each stretch for 20.

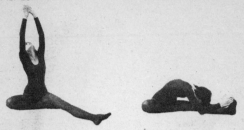

side raise
(24) special techniques

Perform 3 times on each side: once in moderate position and twice in your extreme position on left side, then same on right side. Hold each raise for 10.

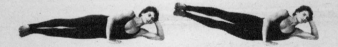

back push-up
(25) special techniques

Perform 3 times: once in the moderate position and twice in your extreme position. Hold each raise for 10.

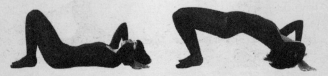

194

shoulder stand
(12) basic techniques

Perform once. Hold for as long as is comfortable. (Remember to raise and lower the legs very slowly to help firm and strengthen legs and abdomen.)

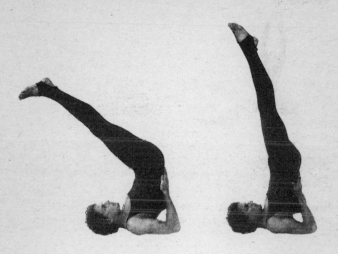

leg over
(23) special techniques

Perform your extreme position 3 times, alternating sides. Hold each for 10.

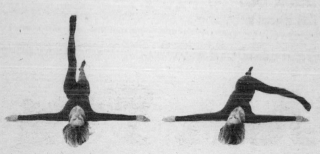

menstruation
(practice during)

This is a highly individual situation for which no specific directions can be offered. Some students are perfectly comfortable in performing their entire **Fitness Program** as usual. Others find that the discomforts of the period can be minimized through a combination of the Shoulder Stand, the mild stretching *asanas* (Back Stretch, Alternate Leg Stretch, Cobra, Chest Expansion), and the breathing techniques (Complete Breath, Alternate Nostril Breathing). Still others perform only Alternate Nostril Breathing and Deep Relaxation. You will have to experiment to determine what is best for you. Whatever you undertake, do it cautiously and intelligently, and attempt to be acutely sensitive to the effect.

pregnancy
(practice during)

With the approval of the physician, the following routine of *asanas* can be performed in the moderate or very elementary positions.

triangle
(4) basic techniques

Perform a moderate position 3 times on each side, alternating sides. Hold each bend for 10.

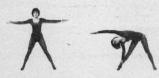

dancer's movements
(6) basic techniques

Perform 5 times. Hold on toes for 5.

back stretch
(7) basic techniques

Perform a moderate position 3 times. Hold each for 10.

alternate leg stretch
(8) basic techniques

Perform a moderate position 3 times with each leg. Hold for 10.

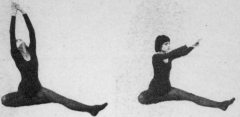

knee and thigh stretch
(9) basic techniques

Perform 3 times. Hold each stretch for 10.

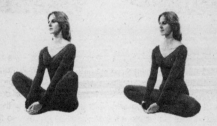

side raise
(24) special techniques

Perform a moderate raise 3 times on each side. Hold each raise for 10.

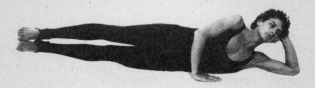

charging breath
(26) special techniques

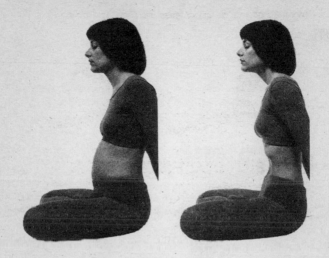

This technique can be very helpful during the final stages of labor. It is similar to the "panting" advocated in various methods of natural childbirth. In a lying position (back or side) you can perform approximately 25 breaths per round and eliminate the Complete Breath that concludes the usual round. Repeat as necessary. Discuss the merits of this technique with your physician during an early stage of pregnancy so that you can perfect the practice well in advance of labor.

Alternate Nostril Breathing (27) Special Techniques and Deep Relaxation (28) Special Techniques will help to relieve discomfort during all stages of pregnancy.

The **Abdomen Routine** is suggested for postnatal practice.

respiration
(nasal, throat, and lung congestion relieved—capacity for deeper breathing increased)

In conjunction with the routine recommended below, strict application of the Yoga nutrition principles—elimination of processed, dairy, and refined-sugar foods, and brief intervals of fasting—are urged. (No improvement in respiratory conditions should be expected if the victim is a smoker.)

charging breath
(26) special techniques

Perform 5 rounds of 25–50 breaths. Follow each round with one Complete Breath. (Coughing, wheezing, and discharge may result from this technique as congestion is loosened.)

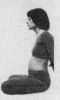 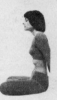

chest expansion
(2) basic techniques; (2A) advanced techniques

Perform twice: once in the moderate position and once in your extreme position. Hold the backward and forward bends for 10 each.

backward bend
(11) basic techniques; (11A) advanced techniques

Perform twice: once in the moderate position and once in your extreme position. Hold each stretch for 20.

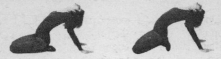

shoulder stand
(12) basic techniques

Perform once. Hold 3 minutes. (Coughing, or a similar effect, may be experienced during or following this inverted position as congestion is loosened.)

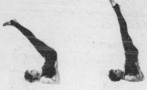

alternate nostril breathing
(27) special techniques

Perform 7 rounds.

When you are entirely comfortable in the Chest Expansion and Backward Bend, you can practice to inhale just prior to the stretch and retain the breath for as long as is comfortable during the actual stretching position. Exhalation can be performed during the **hold** or as you are coming out of the stretch. Retention of the breath can increase the effectiveness of these two *asanas*.

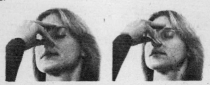

smoking

When the body begins to experience the cleansing and general sense of well-being resulting from the Yoga physical techniques and diet, it frequently loses the desire for cigarettes and, indeed, is even revolted by the odor of the smoke it previously craved. In other words, it becomes clear to you, in a very direct way, that the elevated state of body and mind achieved through the Yoga practice session is immediately eroded by the smoking of a cigarette. At this point, smoking can be naturally abandoned without any special effort of will; you shy away from cigarettes as you would from any noxious substance.

If, during the initial period of abstention from cigarettes, the craving periodically returns, the consciousness can be helped to transcend the desire through seven rounds of Alternate Nostril Breathing (27, Special Techniques).

Remember that a diet which is free of caffeine, flesh products, refined sugar, and processed foods is a great aid in reducing the desire for nicotine.

tension
(physical and emotional relief)

Physical tension occurs at various points in the body where there is tightness, stiffness, or squeezing through muscular contractions that are usually unconscious. Emotional and mental tension result from varying degrees of anxiety and are also a form of tightness or contraction. The solution to these tensions is **decontracting**—releasing what is being held, letting go and relaxing physically, emotionally, and mentally. This decontraction is accomplished through the following routine that is almost immediate in its effect. The entire routine requires approximately fifteen minutes.

chest expansion
(2) basic techniques; (2A) advanced techniques

Perform twice: once in the moderate position and once in your extreme position. Hold the backward bends for 5 and the forward bends for 10.

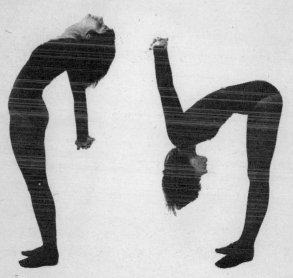

cobra
(14) basic techniques

Perform twice: once in the moderate position and once in your extreme position. Hold each raise for 20.

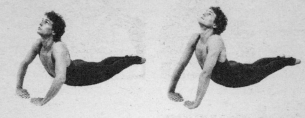

neck movements
(15) basic techniques

Perform the 3 movements twice. Hold each position for 10.

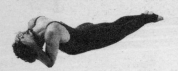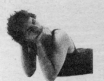

shoulder stand
(12) basic techniques

Perform once. Hold 1–3 minutes.

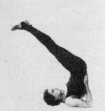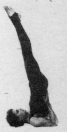

alternate nostril breathing
(27) special techniques

Perform 7 rounds.

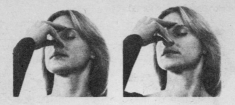

deep relaxation
(28) special technique.

Perform as indicated in the directions.

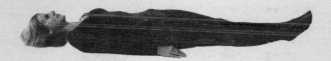

direction of the life-force
(29) special techniques

When the body is in the deeply relaxed state through the previous technique, direct the white light into the forehead. Perform 7 times. Upon completion, lie quietly for as long as is desired.

The regular practice of the **Fitness Program** will assist in preventing tension.

weight regulation and control

The **Fitness Program,** in conjunction with the Yoga diet, will enable many students to accomplish their weight control objectives. If, after working with the **Fitness Program** and applying the nutrition principles for a reasonable period you feel that progress in resolving an excess weight problem is unsatisfactory and that you require a more intensive physical program, you should add to the fitness techniques the various *asanas* contained in the **Abdomen** and **Legs Routines.**

If, subsequent to the more extended practice recommended above, you feel that you require an even more comprehensive plan, we suggest you obtain the *Weight Control Through Yoga* book. This is the same book we have previously recommended for the nutrition and diet information therein.*

*Weight Control Through Yoga, Richard Hittleman, Bantam Books, 1971.

ABOUT THE AUTHOR

RICHARD HITTLEMAN is the world's most widely read author on the subject of Yoga. Born in New York City and introduced to Yoga as a child by a Hindu employee of his parents, Mr. Hittleman became fascinated with the subject and continued its practice throughout his school years. After receiving his masters degree from Columbia University, he embarked upon extensive travel for the purpose of studying Yoga and related oriental disciplines. He began instructing Yoga in the early 1950s. His *Yoga for Health* programs, televised continuously since 1961, are seen throughout the United States and in many foreign countries. He is the author of several books, including *Richard Hittleman's Introduction to Yoga, Richard Hittleman's Guide to Yoga Meditation, Richard Hittleman's Yoga 28 Day Exercise Plan,* and *Weight Control Through Yoga.* During the past twenty-five years, his books, recordings, and instructional albums have enabled millions of people to develop and maintain a high level of physical and mental fitness. Mr. Hittleman lives with his family on the coast of Northern California where he conducts intensive Yoga Workshops several times each year.

Richard Hittleman's *Yoga For Health* television series can be seen in many areas of the country. Information regarding his instructional recordings and Workshops may be obtained from:

YOGA FOR HEALTH
P.O. Box 475
Carmel, CA 93921

BE A WINNER
IN THE RACE FOR
FITNESS

These physical fitness titles give every member of the family the guidance they need for getting in shape and keeping fit. Choose the program most suited to you whether it be yoga, jogging, or an exercise routine. You'll feel better for it.